8-97

OXFORD MEDICAL

THE FACTS

ALSO PUBLISHED BY OXFORD UNIVERSITY PRESS

Panic Disorder

THE FACTS

STANLEY RACHMAN

*Psychology Department, University of
British Columbia, Vancouver*

AND

PADMAL DE SILVA

*Institute of Psychiatry, University of London
Maudsley and Bethlem National Health Service Trust, London*

Oxford   New York   Tokyo
OXFORD UNIVERSITY PRESS

Oxford University Press, Great Clarendon Street, Oxford OX2 6DP

Oxford New York
Athens Auckland Bangkok Bogota Bombay Buenos Aires
Calcutta Cape Town Dar es Salaam Delhi Florence Hong Kong Istanbul
Karachi Kuala Lumpur Madras Madrid Melbourne Mexico City
Nairobi Paris Singapore Taipei Tokyo Toronto Warsaw

and associated companies in
Berlin Ibadan

Oxford is a trade mark of Oxford University Press

Published in the United States
by Oxford University Press Inc., New York

© *Stanley Rachman and Padmal de Silva, 1996*

First published 1996
Reprinted 1998

A catalogue record for this book is available from the British Library

Library of Congress Cataloging in Publication Data
Rachman, Stanley.
Panic disorder / Stanley Rachman and Padmal de Silva.
(Oxford medical publications) (The Facts)
Includes index.
1. Panic disorders. I. De Silva, Padmal. II. Title
III. Series. IV. Series: Facts (Oxford, England)
RC535.R267 1996   616.85'223–dc20   96–2511   CIP

ISBN 0 19 262738 4

Printed in Great Britain on acid-free paper by
Biddles Ltd, Guildford and King's Lynn

Preface

••

This book is intended to provide the reader with basic information about panic disorder, which is relatively common. In our clinical practice we have found the need for a reliable book to recommend to sufferers and their families and friends. We hope that this book will also be of interest to the general reader.

There has been much theoretical and clinical interest in panic disorder in the last twenty years or so, and we have tried to summarize this, and its relevance to patients today. We also give practical advice. References are provided for readers who may wish to read more widely. Research into panic disorder is continuing, and we await new developments and new findings.

Vancouver and   S. R.
London   P. de S.
February 1996

Acknowledgements

· ·

We wish to express our gratitude to Holly Jeffares, Gail Millard, and Christine Lewington who gave excellent secretarial help. We are grateful to the staff of the Oxford University Press who gave valuable editorial advice at various stages. We also thank the authors and publishers who kindly permitted us to quote from their publications.

Contents

• •

1 *Panic and panic disorder*

What is panic?

The term 'panic' is derived from the name of the Greek god Pan. According to Greek mythology, the cloven-footed, dwarfish Pan was a lonely and moody god. He had an impish sense of humour and played practical jokes on humans. If a wanderer happened to pass the cave where he was hiding, Pan would jump out with a shrill and terrifying scream. The acute terror felt by the wanderers who experienced this treatment came to be called 'panic.' A panic is now defined as an episode of intense fear of sudden onset, usually peaking within a minute. The fear, often bordering on terror, is generally accompanied by unpleasant bodily sensations, difficulty in reasoning, and a feeling of imminent catastrophe which can be expressed as: 'Something terrible is happening to me'; 'I am in great danger'.

Some panics are unexpected; it feels as if they 'come out of the blue'. Others are regularly provoked by exposure to identifiable stresses, and therefore can be anticipated. Whether spontaneous or predictable, panics are very upsetting, as shown by the experiences related below.

A 23-year-old woman described her first, unexpected episode of panic: 'I was at home one weekend and suddenly had trouble with my breathing. My heart was pounding and I began sweating heavily. I thought that my heart had given in and felt I was about to die. My husband rushed me to the hospital emergency where they tested my heart and assured me that there was no danger. I gradually calmed down and returned home after an hour or so, feeling shaken but no longer terrified'.

An anxious young accountant, with a long history of worries about her health, nearly choked when a piece of meat was briefly lodged in her throat. She was terrified that she was about to choke to death, remained frightened and upset for an hour or more after the meat was dislodged. Because of her fear of choking, she limited herself from then on to a very narrow, strict diet of soft and easily swallowed foods. Even so, the occasionally felt that some food had not gone down smoothly and would then panic. These panics were always provoked by the same, easily recognized event, enabling her to predict which foods and situations would provoke a panic, and hence avoid them.

A physically active security guard aged 32 experienced his first panic while exercising in a gym. During his usual exercises programme he suddenly became extremely worried about his rapid heart beats; he felt they signalled an imminent heart attack. Understandably, he became frightened and, gasping for air, asked a friend to call for an ambulance. He was rushed to the emergency room of the local hospital, feeling on the trip that he might die before reaching help. He was immediately wheeled into the examination room on arrival. No evidence of any cardiac irregularity or other problem was found, and he was assured that he was healthy and could return home, which he did after resting at the hospital for an hour. Two weeks later he had another unexpected panic while jogging, and again the doctors at the hospital reassured him about his health. A full examination carried out by his family doctor on the following day led to the diagnosis of a panic disorder, and he was referred for psychological treatment.

A 26-year-old woman had a serious car accident while driving with her young child. Although neither was injured, she was very upset by the event. Several weeks later, she had a severe panic attack while driving on her own, and had to pull off the road; she could not continue with her journey. She was terrified by this, her first attack, which was followed by other frequent panics while driving. By the time she was referred to a specialist service she had stopped driving altogether.

A female undergraduate student suddenly began to feel weak in a crowded lecture theatre. She thought she was going to faint, although she had never fainted before, and fearing that she might lose control, quickly found an exit and left the lecture theatre. She felt relieved once outside, but subsequently began to have similar panics in comparably crowded rooms. These situations made her think, 'I will faint', 'I'm going to lose control'. When she was referred for help, she had totally stopped going to classes and other crowded places.

• •

On average, episodes of panic last between 10 and 20 minutes, are extremely distressing, and leave the person feeling drained and apprehensive. Most people experience an occasional episode of panic in which the cause of the fear is evident. The threat of a serious motor accident can provoke it, as can an attack by a vicious dog, and so forth. These panics also are distressing and share some features of the unexpected panics, but at least they are easily understandable. In contrast, the episodes of panic that occur unexpectedly and for no clear reason, are bewildering and therefore, especially troubling. Panics that occur 'out of the blue', unpredictably and inexplicably, are a central feature of 'panic disorder'. Before turning to these disorders, it should be emphasized that most people experience occasional episodes of panic during their lives, which are not necessarily a sign of a psychological disorder.

Panic disorder

In the widely used and comprehensive classification of psychological disorders set out by the American Psychiatric Association, the defining features of panic disorder are given as follows:

1. The person has repeatedly experienced unexpected episodes of panic.

2. In addition, at least one of the episodes was followed by persistent worries, lasting a month or more, of having another panic or about the possible consequences of the attack, or by a significant change in the lifestyle or behaviour related to the panic attacks.

3. During the episodes, at least four of the following sensations/feelings were experienced: shortness of breath, dizziness or faintness, increased heart rate or pounding heart, trembling or shaking, feeling of choking, sweating, stomach distress or nausea, feeling that one's surroundings or oneself are not quite real, feelings of numbness or tingling sensations, hot flushes or chills, chest pain or discomfort, a fear of dying, and a fear of losing control or of going crazy.

4. These attacks are not directly caused by a drug or a general medical condition.

In cases of panic disorder, the episodes may occur as often as daily, or several times per week. After the first episode of unexpected, inexplicable panic, medical reassurance is usually sufficient to provide temporary relief and a sense of calm. However, when the second or subsequent episodes occur, conventional reassurance is of limited value. The person begins to fear that more episodes will take place, and at unpredictable times and in any setting. He/she then becomes anxious and apprehensive, and rarely achieves a satisfactory sense of safety.

Panic disorder with agoraphobia

In a majority of cases, the occurrence of repeated panics is followed by restrictions of the person's regular activities. They tend to avoid situations in which they fear that a panic may occur and/or situations from which a rapid escape might be difficult, including supermarkets, theatres, cinemas, public transport, driving unaccompanied, bridges, or tunnels. Travel by underground train tends to be particularly worrying, as does being caught in a traffic jam or standing in a long line of people. In many instances the affected person becomes fearful even of being alone at home without the reassuring presence of a trusted person who can provide safety (such as by calling a doctor or an ambulance) if a catastrophe threatens. If these fears and the consequent avoidance of 'unsafe' places become excessive, the diagnosis of panic disorder is expanded to 'panic disorder with agoraphobia'. The term 'agoraphobia' strictly means 'fear of the marketplace' but is now generally used to refer to a fear of being in public places from which escape may be difficult, or a fear of coming to harm when alone in one's own home.

Depending on the person's particular fears, the avoidance of 'unsafe' situations may be focused on one or a few places or, in severe cases, extend to virtually any place other than one's house, the company of a few trusted people, or hospitals. In these severe cases the person becomes virtually housebound, unable to travel anywhere alone, and even when accompanied by a trusted adult, can travel for only short distances using specific routes, at specific times.

Anxiety disorders

Panic disorder, with or without agoraphobia, is classified as a form of anxiety disorder, a broad category that includes all forms of psychological disorder in which anxiety is a central feature. The anxiety disorders include 'social phobias', in which the person experiences persistent anxiety in social situations especially if exposed to the scrutiny of others, and 'specific phobias' in which the central feature is an extremely intense, persistent, circumscribed fear of a specific object or place (such as an extreme fear of spiders, or heights). 'Obsessive–compulsive disorder' consists of repetitive, intentional, stereotyped acts, such as compulsive hand washing, and/or repetitive, unwanted, intrusive thoughts of an unacceptable/repugnant quality, and which the affected person resists (see the book by de Silva and Rachman in

Table 1 Anxiety disorders

- Panic disorder, with or without agoraphobia
- Agoraphobia without a history of panics
- Social phobia
- Specific phobia
- Generalized anxiety disorder
- Obsessive–compulsive disorder
- Post-traumatic stress disorder

this series; see p. 94 for reference). 'Post-traumatic stress disorder' is characterized by intense fears that arise and persist after an unusually distressing experience, such as a natural disaster, an accident, or a violent attack. The fears are accompanied by heightened levels of arousal, an involuntary tendency to recall or re-experience the event during dreams or at other times, and by strong tendencies to avoid people or places that are associated with the original stress. 'Generalized anxiety disorder' is characterised by persistent, excessive, unrealistic anxiety about possible misfortunes, such as serious financial losses, ill-health, the welfare of one's children, or combinations of these misfortunes. The category of anxiety disorders is given in Table 1.

Mood disorders

Mood disorders are severe disturbances of mood that are persistent or recurrent. The main disorder is depression in which the person feels unremittingly sad and hopeless/ helpless and experiences a number of accompanying bodily symptoms such as loss of energy, loss of weight, insomnia, and restlessness. Mania is diagnosed if the person experiences episodes of highly elevated mood, abnormal euphoria, overactivity, irritability, loss of judgement, etc. Some patients have alternating depression and mania. They are diagnosed as suffering from bipolar mood disorder or manic-depressive disorder. Of the mood disorders, it is depression that is often found in those with panic disorder. The combination of depression and panic disorder is very debilitating. In some people, the depression relates to the way in which the panic disorder interferes with one's life; in others, the depression is caused by factors unrelated to the panic disorder. The former type of depression tends to go away when the panic is treated; the latter often requires independent treatment.

A note on history

Panic disorder is not a new form of human experience. What is new is its recognition as a separate and identifiable psychological disorder. Although panic disorder was officially recognized as a separate psychiatric category only in 1980 (see Chapter 5), medical authorities had recognized and described panic attacks for a long time previously. For example, a British physician named Hope, in his textbook on cardiology published in 1832, wrote a clear and graphic description of panic, although the word 'panic' was not used. Since the middle of the nineteenth century, physicians have provided descriptions of patients who experienced panic, most of whom were referred to cardiologists. Many of the patients described in this way were soldiers who had experienced war trauma. The recognition that many of these experiences had no physical basis came only later.

2 *The experience of panic*

The main features

Panic is a distressing episode of intense fear during which the person feels that a catastrophe is about to happen—they are dying, losing all control, going insane, or losing consciousness. Although the average duration of panic attack is between 10 and 20 minutes, at the time it seems to be endless. It is perfectly understandable to feel intensely frightened if you believe that you are about to die, which is a common thought in panic episodes. Moreover, the ability to reason is disrupted during panic. Patients say: 'My mind goes blank', 'I feel totally helpless', 'I can't think straight'. Facts that ordinarily would signify safety are difficult to recall or fail to provide the usual reassurance. For example, patients who experience tightness and pain in the chest interpret this as a sign of an impending heart attack despite the fact that repeated medical tests have proved that their cardiac system is entirely normal. One patient said: 'At the time of the panic, I am *convinced* that my heart is giving in even though at other times I know that I've repeatedly been given a clean bill of health'. The most common thoughts experienced during panic have been compiled by Dr Diane Chambless and her colleagues of the Temple University in Philadelphia, and are reproduced in Table 2, listed from the most commonly occurring thought to the least common.

Many physical sensations are associated with panic. The common and intense bodily sensations experienced during panic are listed in Table 3. Of these, the five most common are rapid heart beat, sweating, dizziness, shortness of breath, and shaking, and the most intensely experienced sensations are rapid heart beat, shaking, and shortness of breath. One patient had such intense sensations of a pounding heart that she sometimes felt her heart would actually burst right through her ribs! During one panic episode her heart rate was observed to increase by more than 25 beats per minute. It is not unusual to see an increase of 20 or more heart beats per minute during a panic (but in some episodes, little or no increase occurs). In a typical episode, people experience several of these bodily sensations, which increase in number

Table 2   Thoughts commonly experienced during panic attacks

I will not be able to control myself.
I am going to act foolish.
I am going to pass out.
I am going to go crazy.
I will be paralysed by fear.
I will have a heart attack.
I am going to scream.
I am going to babble or talk funny.
I am going to have a stroke.
I am going to throw up.

From Chambless, Caputo, Bright, and Gallagher (1984). See p. 95 for reference. Reproduced with permission.

Table 3   Common bodily sensations experienced during panic attacks

---

Rapid heart beat
Dizziness
Sweating
Shortness of breath
Shaking
Hot or cold flushes
Chest pain
Faintness
Choking
Feelings of numbness

From Barlow and Craske (1988). See p. 95 for reference. Reproduced with permission.

during intense panics. In a really bad episode they can feel flooded by a rush of disturbing sensations, thereby intensifying the threat of losing control. The sensations are intrusive and they block calm and rational thinking about the true threat, if any. After being buffeted by these disturbing sensations and frightening thoughts, the person may be left anxious, shaken, even exhausted, for between 30 minutes and several hours.

Episodes of panic leave a residue of anxiety long after the attack is over.

Feeling trapped

During panics most people experience a feeling of being *trapped* and their overwhelming thought and need is to escape. This powerful urge to flee can lead to impulsive, risky behaviour, such as driving too fast or recklessly, or dashing blindly out of a building. A patient who had experienced many panics became so apprehensive about panicking when driving her car that she began driving very slowly, and only in the early or late hours of the day. Whenever she sensed the possible onset of a panic she stopped the car regardless of the following traffic. Experiences of this kind result in the avoidance of any similarly threatening situations. In the absence of any change in the occurrence of panics, patients keep adding to their list of places and situations to avoid, and in extreme cases become as housebound as people with major physical disabilities. Since they appear fit and healthy, their inability to leave the home can be puzzling to relatives and friends.

The first panic

Roughly one-third of the initial panics occur in public places, about one-quarter start while driving or being driven in a car, and one-third begin at home. In most cases it is possible to identify a major source of stress at or shortly before the first panic (such as personal conflicts, work stress, personal loss or grief, birth/pregnancy). The person's interpretation of and reaction to that first panic depends on the accompanying bodily sensations and the circumstances of the panic. A common example is an unexpected panic which features rapid heart beats, shortness of breath, and a sense of great danger. This is commonly interpreted as the start of a heart attack (or other medical catastrophe) and the person is taken to an emergency medical service. When the doctors conclude that the person's cardiac system is functioning normally, the person immediately feels relieved. However, it leaves unexplained the nature and cause of the discomfort and distress, and the absence of a satisfactory explanation is a breeding ground for anxiety.

When a second episode occurs and the doctors again confirm the absence of any cardiac or other medical problem, some patients begin to doubt their sanity. The episodes of anxiety are distressing and accompanied by intense bodily sensations that are undeniable and uncontrollable. But, so the reasoning goes, 'there is nothing medically wrong with me,' 'yet I certainly am not imagining all this, nor making it up, and it is totally out of control. Am I perhaps going crazy?' More accurately, the patient could conclude that there is nothing wrong with the cardiac system, but that they now have a problem of episodically uncontrollable anxiety—a problem as real and distressing as any physical problem. Regrettably, anxiety problems are less well understood, and hence less well tolerated by family, friends, and employers. Usually after the first panic, but certainly after subsequent panics, the person becomes extremely anxious and apprehensive. Additionally, he/she may become restless, irritable and pre-occupied with the problem. Once the person is persuaded by repeated medical reassurance that there is no danger of an imminent medical catastrophe, their anxiety may be focused on the danger of another panic. They begin to fear the panic itself—a fear of fear. Accordingly, when they anticipate having a panic they engage in strict avoidance of any places where a panic may be embarrassing or humiliating. The following case illustrates this.

The first panic of Mr J., a 31-year-old shopkeeper, was provoked by a feeling of tightness in the chest accompanied by rapid breathing, which he took to mean that he was about to have a heart attack. After two more episodes, and extensive medical examinations, he was convinced that his health was, after all, sound. However, he now developed a fear of having panics, particularly as he felt out of control during those episodes. As a result he avoided driving or walking over bridges, driving on highways, and so forth, because he was frightened of having a panic, losing control of himself and causing an accident. In many cases of panic disorder, the original fear of physical harm is replaced by a fear of loss of control or social embarrassment. Most often, the original fear is gradually replaced by the fear of having an episode of panic. For example, 'I dare not travel alone because I may have one of my panics'.

Unexpected panics

The most puzzling, and probably the most disruptive, panics are those that occur unexpectedly, out of the blue. We have no trouble in understanding a panic that occurs in reaction to an obvious and predictable danger situation such as parachuting out of an aircraft, but the panics that take place while sitting quietly at home are difficult to explain. There is no external threat and no reason to anticipate any threat, but with little warning the person begins to sweat, is short of breath, and has a pounding heart. Often these sensations are interpreted as signs of some internal threat, some danger to one's health. In the absence of any good explanation for the panic, it is virtually impossible to predict when and where the next episode will occur. The unpredictable and inexplicable qualities of these panics are an added worry and burden. As one cannot be fully assured of being safe at any time or place, it becomes difficult to plan activities.

With repeated episodes, it is possible to identify triggers for the unexpected panics, and detect some pattern in their occurrence. As will be seen in Chapter 4, the psychological consequences of unexpected panics are more serious and disruptive than those that follow predictable panics.

The occurrence of at least some unexpected panics is regarded as a diagnostic sign of a panic disorder.

Situational panics

Most panics occur in response to some perceived external threat, such as being enclosed in a small room. These situational panics share most of the features of unexpected panics, but are more predictable, and hence easier to avoid, than the unexpected variety. Situational panics tend to occur directly on exposure to the threatening situation, but the response is occasionally delayed. Strong anticipation of such an exposure can also cause a panic. Situational panics occur in virtually all cases of panic disorder, and are also very common in most of the other anxiety disorders.

Nocturnal panics

Some people who experience episodes of panic are also affected by occasional panics during the early hours of sleep. Typically, the person wakes up in a state of panic. Studies suggest that about one-quarter of all people with panic disorder have had this experience. Nocturnal panics share most of the characteristics of ordinary panics, including rapid heart beats and shortness of breath, plus rather more sensations of choking. In roughly half of nocturnal panics, patients report that their first symptom upon awakening is a fearful thought such as dying or losing control, and in the remaining half, the first symptom is a bodily sensation such as choking. Nocturnal panics tend to be severe and last for roughly 25 minutes on average, although the duration can vary. Some people report very brief nocturnal panic attacks, lasting for one or two minutes, while others report a long duration. Nocturnal panics do not appear to be triggered by bad dreams and, unlike some other nocturnal disorders, panics are not accompanied by any disturbance of consciousness. During a nocturnal panic the person is normally responsive and attentive, and later can recall the event without difficulty.

Relaxation-induced panics

In most circumstances fear and relaxation have opposite effects, and as a result relaxation techniques are a valuable and widely used means of reducing or blocking fear. However, in a small number of panic cases, the onset of relaxation actually triggers a panic. A 25-year-old woman who had experienced a bad reaction to a 'street' drug, which made her feel like she was drifting out of control, possibly to her death, developed a fear and avoidance of medications. She also had a panicky reaction to relaxation training because the spreading sensations of muscle relaxation re-evoked the sense of losing control and the threat of death.

These relaxation-induced panics generally arise from an intense fear of losing control. It is also possible that, in attempting to relax, their attention is drawn to bodily sensations about which they are already anxious; a further possibility is that relaxation reduces normal barriers to worrisome thoughts. Patients who tend to have panics during relaxation require a modified form of conventional treatment that excludes relaxation training unless special care is taken to overcome the person's reaction. In such cases, techniques of relaxation focusing more on imagery may be used.

3 Facts about panic

Frequency

Many people experience the occasional panic, without adverse or long-term consequences, particularly if the episode can be explained by an identifiable external threat, and is not unexpected. They have more difficulty coping with panics that come 'out of the blue', hence the importance which clinicians attach to severe, unexpected panics. Among the general population up to one-third of people report having had at least one panic in the past year, but the panics tend to be less severe as well as less frequent than those associated with panic disorder. Having an occasional episode of panic is common and not a sign of any psychological disorder.

Panic and agoraphobia

Panic with agoraphobia is the combination of distressing episodes of sudden, intense fear, plus the disabling fear and avoidance of particular places/activities. It is extremely unusual for agoraphobia to develop in the absence of a history of panics, although it occasionally does and this is recognized in diagnostic schemes (see Table 1, p.5).

The most common consequence of repeated panics is the apprehensive avoidance of places or activities that have become associated with panic. People also tend to avoid situations from which easy, rapid escape might be difficult in the event of a panic (such as sitting in the centre row of a theatre, travelling by underground train). Agoraphobia was originally believed to be a fear of open spaces, but the fear and avoidance generally are more extensive than this. Prior to the introduction of the diagnosis of panic disorder, most patients who feared and avoided public and other places were given the diagnosis of agoraphobia, and panic episodes were regarded as incidental. The places usually avoided in agoraphobia are public transport, enclosed spaces such as tunnels, bridges, slowed traffic, supermarkets, queues, and travelling long distances from home. Various activities, such as vigorous exercise or drinking coffee, can provoke anxiety, and are therefore avoided.

When the person is unable to avoid an anxiety-arousing place or situation, as in an unexpected traffic jam, he/she feels trapped and experiences an overwhelming urge to leave, to flee.

With their mobility and activities restricted, affected people are obliged to make numerous changes in their daily lives. Most sufferers find that the restrictions are eased somewhat when they are accompanied by a trusted adult; they can travel a little further (for example, carry out the shopping if accompanied). Patients who are taking tranquillizing medications generally feel that their mobility is slightly expanded when they are medicated. There is also some variation in their mobility, dependent on mood: on a 'good' day the person may be able to use a bus, but on a 'bad' day have difficulty even leaving the house.

Panic episodes in other anxiety disorders

The original notion that episodes of panic are a feature distinctive of panic disorder has been replaced by a recognition that occasional panics occur in the general population, and that in various forms of anxiety disorder, panics are extremely common. Panics are almost as common in social phobias, obsessive–compulsive disorder, generalized anxiety disorder and specific phobias as they are in panic disorder. It is not uncommon for a social phobic patient to experience panic even at the thought of speaking before a group of people. Panics are also common in depression. However, in panic disorder the episodes tend to be more severe, more frequent, and more unpredictable, than they are in other forms of anxiety disorders or in depression.

What precipitates a panic disorder?

Most panic disorders appear to be brought on by a stressful event or period. Given the unexpected onset of the first few panics, many patients are at a loss to explain their sudden experience of intense fear. However, during assessment and treatment, the stressful trigger of the panic tends to emerge.

Major changes in one's life can bring on panics, and the most common triggers are: marital/personal conflict, illness or death of a close person, births or miscarriages, and financial threats or loss. Stress at work, health problems, and negative reactions to drugs are also known to increase the risk of triggering a panic. The fact that most people endure these negative events without panicking points to the existence of some risk factors that make some people especially vulnerable to episodes of panic.

● ●

Mr T., a successful and busy accountant, was a chronic worrier and easily discouraged. His mother developed a serious incapacitating illness which required him to visit her frequently and to oversee her health and other needs. Soon after, his first panic episodes began, which were unexpected and extremely frightening. On more than one occasion he felt like he was going to die. Initially, Mr T. did not connect the stress of coping with his mother's illness to his panics, which he regarded as an added but independent problem. Later, he described how distressed and over-stretched he had been feeling immediately prior to his first panic. Additionally, his mother's illness had provoked intense fears of his own mortality.

Ms C.'s first episode of panic was precipitated by a bad reaction to smoking cannabis. She began to feel extremely light-headed, out of control, and dizzy, and that her surroundings were unreal. She thought she was going completely insane and became terrified. This initial episode was followed by prolonged anxiety and she became acutely sensitive to unusual tastes or odours. Whenever she felt light-headed or unreal, her anxiety increased and on many occasions she had full panics.

● ●

Risk factors

Research into the factors that contribute to the risk of developing a panic disorder is relatively recent and incomplete. However, in recent research from South Carolina the following risk factors were identified: family conflict, lack of parental support, separation anxiety during childhood, chronic physical or psychiatric illness in the family, and the abuse of alcohol or drugs in the family. There was no evidence that parental death, divorce, or sexual abuse were risk factors for panic disorder. Independent research on respiratory illnesses indicates that people who have a history of difficulties with their breathing are at increased risk for panic disorder.

Genetics

There appears to be a slightly increased risk of panic disorder among people who are born into families in which a close relative has had a diagnosed panic disorder. It is not yet known for certain whether this is because of genetic factors or as a result of their contact with the sufferer. The evidence of panic disorder among sets of identical twins and sets of non-identical twins, which would help to identify a genetic contribution to the disorder, is too sparse to help clear up this point. Genetic factors appear to play a small but significant role in increasing a person's vulnerability to various forms of anxiety disorder, such as obsessive – compulsive disorder. The same may well be true for panic disorder.

Separation anxiety

There is conflicting evidence on whether or not separation anxiety in childhood predisposes people to panic disorders in later life. The term 'separation anxiety' refers to the distress exhibited by young children provoked by separation from a parent, usually the mother. Some people with panic disorder report that they had separation anxiety but the findings, based as they are on the person's recall of childhood events and feelings, are not reliable. The majority of children who experience prolonged separations do so without ill effects.

The size of the problem

Roughly 15 people per 1000 in the general population develop a panic disorder at some time in their life. The size of the problem is much the same from country to country, and no ethnic or racial differences have been found. Roughly comparable figures have been reported from different countries—e.g., Canada, Italy, Korea, New Zealand, and the United States.

Persistent panic disorder has an adverse effect on most aspects of the person's life—marital relationship, mobility, social contacts, employment, economic status. It can be extremely disabling. There is very little information about the natural course of (untreated) panic disorder, but the long term results of a large study of the effects of anti-panic medications provide a rough guide to the outcome of the disorder. Half of the patients showed recurrent or mild symptoms, 30% recovered, and in 20% of the cases panic disorder followed a severe, chronic course. Psychological treatment is effective in a majority of cases, but the long-term effects are yet to be clarified.

Age and sex

It is rare for the onset of panic disorder to occur before the age of 15, although there are occasional cases in childhood (see below). The onset in the majority of cases occurs in the twenties. In this sense, it is a disorder of early adulthood. The chances of someone developing panic disorder for the first time after the age of 40 are slim. The disorder is roughly twice as frequent in the 25–44 age range as it is in the 45–64-year-old group. Panic disorder is infrequent in people over 65 years old.

The sex distribution is also uneven. In most studies, there are more females patients than males, mainly because there are more females who have panic disorder with agoraphobia. In this group, the female to male ratio is about 3:1. This may, of course, be at least partly due to societal expectations and stereotypes. It has been suggested that females may tend to deal with anticipatory anxiety and fear of panic by avoiding the situations associated with panic attacks, leading to agoraphobia, whereas males may force themselves to confront these situations, possibly with the help of alochol or drugs. Among panic disorder patients without agoraphobia, the sex difference is less marked.

Relation of panic disorder to other disorders

Roughly half of diagnosed panic disorder patients have been clinically depressed at some time in their lives. Approximately one-quarter have suffered from a social phobia at some time, and the same proportion have had obsessive–compulsive problems. About one in five has abused alcohol.

At the time of diagnosis, many panic disorder patients are also found to have other psychological problems. Roughly 40% have depression concurrent with the panic disorder, and it is not clear whether the depressive symptoms in these cases should be seen as an independent disorder, or a result of the restrictions and misery caused by the panic disorder. The other disorders commonly associated with panic disorder at diagnosis include social phobia and hypochondriasis. Hypochondriasis is a condition in which the predominant disturbance is groundless anxiety concerning health—either the fear of having, or the belief that one has, a serious physical illness. A related problem associated with panic disorder is what has been called 'somatization disorder'. This is characterized by recurrent and multiple physical complaints of several years' duration, for which medical help is sought but which are not due to any physical disorder. It generally begins before the age of 30, and has a chronic and fluctuating course. A proportion of these patients have been shown to suffer from panic disorder. In one American study, over a half of the patients with somatization disorder were found to satisfy all the diagnostic criteria for panic disorder. As many panic patients tend to complain, understandably, about their physical symptoms, such as shortness of breath, palpitations, and chest pain, it is likely that the true nature of their disorder is not detected early by doctors in many cases. So they spend many years seeking help for the physical symptoms.

Panic in children

Panic disorder is rarely diagnosed in children, but a small number of children and young adolescents do have panic episodes which do not differ from those in adults. Indeed, a small but significant proportion of adult patients with panic disorder report an onset before the age of 10. Several recent studies have provided evidence of panic disorder among children referred for psychological or psychiatric help; for example, some children presenting with school phobia or school refusal have been shown to have frequent panic episodes in school settings.

• •

Anna was referred for help at the age of 12. The picture presented was one of general anxiety and school refusal. During careful assessment, it emerged that Anna had typical panic disorder. She had her first panic episode at the age of eight when, in the presence of many other children, she was severely reprimanded by a teacher for being late. She then began to have panics in the school assembly, in the playground when surrounded by other children, and occasionally on her way to school. She had been taken to various medical experts before persistent school refusal led to her being referred to a psychological service.

Anna described her panic attacks as involving feelings of weakness, pounding heart, trembling, dizziness, shortness of breath, and a fear that she might die. Most of her panics had occurred in or near the school premises, although she also had occasional panics in other places.

• •

Cases have also been found of children developing panic problems in the context of war and related to being subjected to violence. While the numbers are relatively small, it is important to recognize these problems when they do occur in children, so that appropriate help can be given.

4 *The consequences of panic*

Most episodes of panic are distressing, but the psychological consequences can be disabling and can persist for years. As described in Chapter 3, after a number of panic episodes, it is likely that the affected person will begin to avoid particular places and activities. This type of avoidance can become so severe as to shape and limit their entire life—personal life, marriage, employment, travel and so on. It can also have a major impact on the person's social life. In extreme cases the person is unable to leave the house except when accompanied, and then only for short distances and brief periods.

The exact pattern of the avoidance behaviour is determined mainly by the person's particular fears. Someone who fears that exertion may bring on a heart attack will, of course, avoid energetic actions such as sports. A person who fears that he/she may lose control and jump off a bridge will avoid bridges and other high places. A person who fears suffocation will avoid tunnels, elevators, tube trains, and so forth.

The main concern behind this avoidance behaviour is to ensure one's safety, and to have easy and rapid access to safety in all potentially risky situations. For example, the person may avoid being alone at home in case of a medical disaster; or travelling alone; or ensure that a car is always available and reliable; that they always sit on the aisle and near an exit; and avoid shopping unaccompanied; avoid waiting in queues; or ensure that the hotel room is on the ground level, and is well-aired.

A list of the most common forms of avoidance is provided in Table 4. This comes from a study carried out by Dr Dianne Chambless and her colleagues, using the Mobility Inventory they developed. The Inventory is reproduced in Appendix 1.

Episodes of panic usually engender feelings of anxious apprehension. It is extremely common to feel anxious for periods each day, accompanied by feelings of restlessness, and irritability. Worry, pre-occupation with the panics and their significance, and feelings of depression are common consequences of panic episodes.

As described in Chapter 1, there is a common transition from the fear of a medical or physical disaster to a fear of having another episode of

Table 4 Common forms of avoidance

Going in airplanes
Being far away from home
Underground and tunnels
Going in ships/boats
Theatres
Going in buses
Going in trains
Museums
Stadiums/auditoriums
High places
Driving on motorways
Department stores
Restaurants
Enclosed spaces
Standing in queues
Parties
Crossing bridges
Supermarkets

From Chambless, Caputo, Jasin, Gracely, and Williams (1985). See p. 95 for reference. Reproduced with permission.

panic. There is a close connection between the person's fear of another panic and particular forms of avoidance; they will strongly avoid any and all situations in which they anticipate that a panic is very likely to occur. One patient said: 'I keep away from the market because I know a panic is certain to occur.' An obvious example is, 'I avoid using elevators because I *know* that I will panic'.

In general, the person's expectation of a panic is the strongest determinant of avoidance on a particular day in a particular place. If they predict that a panic is highly likely, the place or event will be avoided. However, if they anticipate that no panic or other disaster will occur in that particular place at that time, then there is no need or urge to avoid.

Most sufferers from panic disorder experience fluctuations in their anxiety and their expectations of panic. They have good days and bad days, and sometimes know on waking what to expect. In part these fluctuations are caused by changes in mood, but it also is possible to make sense of many fluctuations by close analysis of the person's thoughts about the possibility of disaster.

The mere fact that the anxiety, expectations of panic, and especially the avoidance behaviour do fluctuate can be a source of misunderstanding and conflict within the family. It is commonly believed that a person's behaviour is, or should be, consistent from day to day. And the ability to travel to work unaccompanied, to take one example, should be consistent. An irate relative who says, 'Why must I travel with you today when you were perfectly capable of going on your own yesterday?' reflects this belief that people should be consistent in their behaviour. To the observer, especially close family members or friends, the variability in the sufferer's avoidance behaviour, and in the demands made upon friends and relatives, is puzzling. The variability sometimes calls into question the authenticity of the sufferer's problems: Are they genuinely panicky? Do they really need me to stay at home with them? Is there perhaps an element of faking or pretending? At other times, the apparently inexplicable fluctuations in the patient's anxiety/avoidance may be mistaken as a sign of deep mental instability.

Many of these doubts and misunderstandings are based on the incorrect assumption that anxiety and avoidance are consistent and unchanging. 'As you were free of anxiety and could travel unimpeded on Tuesday, you should be able to do the same on Friday'. In fact, anxiety does fluctuate a good deal, and the fearful anticipation of having a panic can vary from one day to the next. The reasons for these fluctuations are seldom obvious even to the sufferer, and add to the irrational quality of panic disorders.

They do have irrational qualities, just as many other fears have an irrational element such as intense fears of harmless spiders. It is important for friends and family to realize that a person who experiences apparently irrational panics is not wholly irrational or mentally unstable. After all, there are irrational features in almost all forms of human behaviour; we all think and behave irrationally at times, without being considered psychologically abnormal.

After a few episodes of panic people begin to make informal predictions about if and when they will experience another panic. After an unexpected panic they are likely to think that the next panic is far more probable than it really is. Such overprediction is very common. Far more episodes of panic are expected than ever occur.

The tendency to expect the worst is, however, modifiable. With repeated experiences of panics and of periods/places free of panic, the sufferer's predictions become more accurate, and they learn to anticipate reasonably well when panics are likely to occur. Just as the predictions of further panics are modifiable, so predictions of a safe period are also modifiable, although it takes many more experiences of safety to reassure the sufferer that a panic is very unlikely to occur. Fear and anxiety are quickly increased by a panic episode, but regaining confidence about one's safety is a considerably slower process. It is a process that can be facilitated by systematic treatment.

5   *Theories of panic disorder*

· ·

There are two main approaches to understanding the causes of panic disorder, one which emphasizes biological factors and the other which emphasizes psychological factors. It is widely agreed that both biological and psychological factors are involved, but opinions differ on the relative importance of each type, and how they combine. At present there is no fully satisfactory and comprehensive explanation of panic disorders, but progress is being made. As with some other medical and psychological problems, the absence of a satisfactory explanation of panic disorder has not precluded the development of effective treatment methods. Therapeutic progress often precedes theoretical explanations.

The biological theory

The occurrence of episodes of panic is not new, but in the 1960s a psychiatrist at the New York Psychiatric Institute, Dr Donald Klein, suggested that people who repeatedly experience severe panics, especially unexpected panics, are suffering from a separate and distinctive disorder: panic disorder. After a good deal of research his suggestion was accepted and the diagnosis of panic disorder was included, in 1980, in the major classification system of the American Psychiatric Association. The classifications are set out in the Association's *Diagnostic and Statistical Manual* (see p. 95 for reference) which has now been adopted in a large number of countries. Dr Klein based his suggestion on two main pieces of evidence. First, he observed that patients who experienced severe, unexpected panics failed to respond to medications that reduced most other types of anxiety disorder, but surprisingly did respond favourably to one drug, imipramine (see p.31), which is used mainly as a treatment for depression. He concluded therefore that the panic sufferers were different from the patients who had other forms of anxiety disorder.

Secondly, many of the panic sufferers in a laboratory test experienced attacks when sodium lactate was infused into them. Fewer patients with other types of anxiety disorder responded in this way to this test, and

Dr Klein used these results to strengthen his suggestion that repeated episodes of panic indicate the presence of a separate and distinctive disorder. Moreover, when panic patients were medicated with the anti-depressant drug imipramine, they were far less likely to have an attack during the laboratory test for panic. Dr Klein concluded that the drug blocked the laboratory panics, which indicated a biological basis for the disorder.

Dr Klein proposed that panic disorders are primarily biological in nature: patients have a super-sensitive alarm system that is repeatedly and unexpectedly triggered by pathological discharges in the nervous system, causing spontaneous panics. These discharges are thought to be linked to fears of suffocation, or of separation anxiety. The spontaneous panics occur at unpredicatable times, including nocturnal panics, and hence can occur in unexpected places. The experience of spontaneous panics gives rise to apprehension about further episodes, increased anxiety, and eventually agoraphobia.

Dr Klein's work has had a wide impact and his main suggestion, that panic disorder is a separate disorder, is generally, though not universally, accepted. In addition, the link between panic and subsequent fear and avoidance has been confirmed.

The theory of a pathological central discharge in the nervous system has fared less well, and indeed Dr Klein has recently revised his original ideas. The problems began when it was found that, contrary to the initial reports, patients with panic disorder did in fact respond favourably to certain drugs that are effective in treating other forms of anxiety disorder. Panic disorders do not after all respond only and distinctively to a particular, anti-depressant drug.

The second plank in Dr Klein's theory, that panic disorder patients respond distinctively and predictably to the sodium lactate laboratory test, was not confirmed. Later research revealed that patients with disorders other than panic disorder, and even some people free of any disorder, can also give similer responses to the test. Furthermore, the original idea that most panic disorder patients have attacks when given sodium lactate had to be revised; the revised estimates were that roughly 50% of panic disorder patients give this response, rather than the 85% or so originally thought to do so. As it was originally believed that the laboratory test is effective because it triggered a central discharge of the over-sensitive alarm system, the growing numbers of different responses among panic disorder patients presented a problem.

It meant that even if the theory were correct, it might apply to only a subset of panic disorder patients. Moreover, the fact that numbers of non-panic disorder patients also gave similar responses to the test had not been predicted.

It was also pointed out that the distinction between the spontaneous panics, to which Dr Klein attached great importance, and the other more common panics, was not as clear as implied in the theory. Critics also complained that the theory was unacceptably vague on significant details.

In a recent revision of the theory, Dr Klein has suggested that we are all equipped with a sensitive, in-born suffocation alarm system. However, if that system is too easily and/or too frequently set-off, it can induce a spontaneous panic. It follows that the underlying problem for many or even most panic disorder sufferers is a super-sensitive suffocation alarm system. Research on this theory has commenced and should bear fruit within a few years. It certainly is the case that many sufferers of panic disorder experience breathing difficulties and that an intense fear of suffocation could be an important factor among these people.

It must be noted that Dr Klein's account is only one of several biological theories of panic disorder. Theorists have put forward different views of a biological cause, with some suggestive evidence. Overall, however, none of these is supported at present by convincing evidence.

Psychological theories

It was indeed the observation of breathing difficulties in panic disorder patients that sparked off what later became one of the most influential alternatives to Dr Klein's biological theory. Like many clinicians before and since, Dr David Clark of Oxford University's Department of Psychiatry noted the frequency with which these patients experience breathing difficulties. Their breathing tends to be too rapid and/or too shallow. The effects of overbreathing (hyperventilation) often include dizziness, feeling light-headed, rapid heart beat, unsteadiness, tingling of the extremities, tightness of the chest, and even a sense of unreality.

Among panic disorder sufferers, many of the episodes of panic are preceded by overbreathing. Dr Clark's observations led him to believe that the panics tend to occur when the person thinks that the effects of overbreathing (such as light-headedness, chest pressure) means that something terrible is about to happen. For example: 'My chest is tight and I feel dizzy and faint, which means I am having a heart attack. I am about to die'. Dr Clark expanded his work beyond the study of overbreathing to include a range of unpleasant and/or unexplained bodily sensations and then constructed a fresh explanation for panic disorder. He suggested that episodes of panic are caused by a catastrophic misinterpretation of various bodily sensations. The person becomes intensely frightened of an immediate danger.

The most common forms of misinterpretation are a fear of imminent death, a fear of going insane, a fear of completely losing control, a fear of public embarrassment/humiliation, and a fear of a brain tumour or other serious disease. People who are predisposed to fear one or more of these personal catastrophes, either because of their personal or family history, and who are acutely sensitive to their bodily sensations, are at increased risk of developing panic disorder.

Any event or situation that provokes unpleasant bodily sensations, such as faintness caused by overbreathing, is open to misinterpretation. A person who is especially frightened of an early death by sudden heart attack, say because of a family history of heart trouble, may misinterpret tightness in his chest when exercising as a symptom of a coming attack, and panic. However, if that same person explains the feeling as a normal response to exercising, then he will not panic.

Where do these catastrophic thoughts come from? In most fully analyzed cases the thoughts are traceable to the sufferer's personal experiences (for example, a history of breathing problems such as asthma, or a life-threatening episode of choking) or to serious illnesses, death, or catastrophes which they have witnessed, or heard about, in close relatives or friends. For example, the patient mentioned on p.53 below was frightened of developing a fatal recurrence of cancer just as her mother and aunt had done. Another patient feared that his occasional feelings of 'unreality' were a sign that he would become schizophrenic and be confined in a long-stay hospital, as had the uncle whom he visited in a psychiatric hospital. These visits, which began when the patient was an adolescent, were always distressing and he was anxiously aware of thinking that he might follow his uncle into insanity.

To summarize: the perception of unpleasant/unexplained bodily sensations provides the opportunity for a fear reaction. If the person makes a catastrophic misinterpretation of the sensations, a panic is likely to follow. If the person places a safe, benign interpretation on the sensations, there will be no panic.

• •

A 25-year-old woman with no history of psychological troubles was voluntarily taking part in a laboratory demonstration of the effects of standing in a small enclosed space (a sort of telephone kiosk in this particular experiment) for up to two minutes. To her surprise she had felt hot and flushed in the enclosed space and begun to sweat profusely, her breathing was rapid and shallow, she had become acutely upset by a feeling of being trapped, and then panicked. Later, she explained that she had thought she was about to faint and completely lose control of herself.

When asked if she had ever experienced similar physical sensations (flushes, sweating, shortness of breath) at other times, she promptly replied that it reminded her of how she felt after jogging. She then added: 'But that has never bothered me because I know that exercise causes sweating and panting'. A benign interpretation of the same physical sensations produced no fear.

• •

Clark and his colleagues were able to show that panic disorder patients not only report lots of spontaneously occurring frightening thoughts, but that if the patients are encouraged to produce the relevant physical sensations (such as overbreathing) and also make a worrying interpretation of the sensations, intense fear follows. It turns out that panic disorder patients, and others who are vulnerable to panic, respond fearfully to purely psychological (behavioural) changes, such as entering a small, enclosed space. So panic can be induced in a proportion of panic disorder patients by biological or by psychological stimulation.

A simple diagram illustrating the cognitive model of panic attacks is given in Figure 1. In Figure 2, a specific example of a patient's panic attack is provided.

Dr Clark's psychological theory, and a similar theory developed independently by Dr David Barlow of the State University of New York at Albany, can account for many aspects of panic disorder, including the previously puzzling fact that some patients experience panics when they begin to feel deeply relaxed. These so-called relaxation panics occur among people who fear a catastrophe, such as death

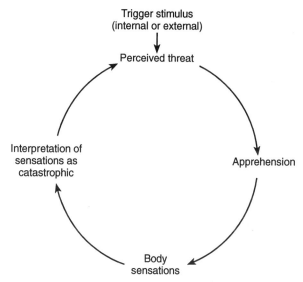

Figure 1 A cognitive model of panic attacks. From Clark (1986). See p.95 for reference. Reproduced with permission.

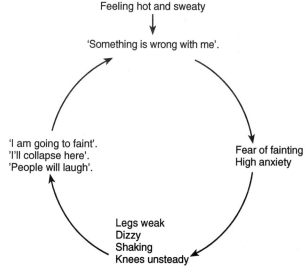

Figure 2 Cognitive model of panic attacks: a specific example.

or insanity, if they totally lose control; they feel they must hold on to their conscious control in all of their waking hours, or else. These fears sometimes have their origin in disturbing experiences with illegal drugs. Not surprisingly, these people are resistant to taking any drugs, even prescribed ones.

The psychological theories have their limitations, and cannot yet explain fully the occurrence of nocturnal panics, and of some of the effects of therapy. As will be described in Chapter 6, the therapy that grew out of the psychological approach is effective, but some forms of psychological therapy that ignore the patient's interpretations of their sensations and thoughts are also effective. The question that then arises is whether the change from misinterpretations to correct interpretations is indeed a necessary part of effective treatment. If improvements occur even without any deliberate attempt to correct the misinterpretations, then such corrections either occur spontaneously or are not necessary for change.

From theory to treatment

Both the biological and psychological theories have been used as a foundation for the development of treatments for panic disorder. The biological approach has spawned a continuous search for effective new drugs, especially those with minimal side-effects. The psychological approach gave rise to cognitive–behavioural therapy, in which patients are guided towards more appropriate interpretations of their experiences, and are taught how to reduce the intensity and frequency of their disturbing bodily sensations. These will be discussed in some detail in Chapters 6 and 7.

For readers who wish to read more detailed accounts of the theories, and critical commentaries on them, some of the key references are given in the annotated reading list provided in Appendix 5.

6 *Treatment of panic disorder*

Developments in treatment

Panic disorder is a treatable condition. There are two effective forms of treatment, psychological therapy and medication. The panel of experts who participated in a consensus conference on the subject organized by the National Institutes of Health of the United States in 1991 concluded that psychological treatments are of 'demonstrated efficacy in the reduction and/or elimination of panic attacks and agoraphobia. Early reports ... indicate that significant numbers of patients are panic-free at the end of ... treatment and remain so at a 2-year follow-up'. The treatment is well tolerated and acceptable to most patients. In addition, three classes of medication 'have been found to be effective in reducing or eliminating panic attacks associated with the various forms of panic disorder' (Wolfe and Maser 1994). Some of the medications tend to produce unwanted side-effects however, and occasionally cause patients to discontinue the treatment.

Medication

As originally described by Dr Klein, the anti-depressant drug imipramine (Janimine, SK-pramine, Tofranil) is a demonstrably effective treatment for panic disorder. Imipramine belongs to the 'tricyclic' group of anti-depressants, so called because of their chemical structure. Imipramine generally blocks the episodes of panic and reduces the patient's general anxiety. Depression, as noted in an earlier chapter, is a common accompaniment of panic disorder and imipramine can serve a double purpose by simultaneously reducing both panic disorder and depression.

The drug is usually given in small doses initially, for example 25 mg, and gradually increased by 25 mg every three days to an average 150 mg per day, over a period of two to three weeks. Many patients require high doses for the drug to be effective, in some cases as high as 300 mg per day. The beneficial effects of the medication tend to appear roughly three to four weeks after treatment begins. Common side-effects are: dry mouth, blurred vision, nausea, light-headedness, urinary retention, constipation, weight gain, overstimulation, drowsiness, postural hypotension, sweating, and sexual difficulties. In most cases, patients become accustomed to the drug and the side-effects tend to diminish. However, between one-quarter and one-third of patients experience intolerable levels of side-effects that lead them to discontinue the medication.

Before starting the medication, patients are prepared by the provision of full information and an explanation of the therapeutic benefits and the expected side-effects.

Patients tend to be kept on the medication for up to 12 months; when the drug is withdrawn, it is done gradually and carefully, usually over a period of three months, in order to avoid withdrawal reactions and/or relapse.

The drug should not be taken by people who have cardiac disorders, mania, urinary difficulties, and glaucoma. Further, imipramine should never be taken at the same time as other anti-depressants, particularly those in MAOI group (see below).

Other tricyclic anti-depressants that have anti-panic effects include clomipramine (Anafranil) and desipramine (Pertofran, Norpramin).

A second type of anti-depressant medication, the monoamine oxidase inhibitors (MAOI), has also been shown to be effective, but is less frequently prescribed because of side-effects, adverse interactions with other medications, and the need to adopt a restrictive diet. The possible side-effects include dry mouth, constipation, blurred vision, postural hypotension, insomnia, sexual problems, and weight gain. It is not suitable for people with blood pressure problems, cardiovascular disorders or headaches, and should not be taken at the same time as other anti-depressants, or with any of a range of other medications. Food or preparations which contain tyramine (including cheese, beer, red wine, and meat extracts) are prohibited. The list of precautions for MAOI drugs is lengthy and extra care must be taken with these prescriptions. The medication is introduced slowly after giving the patient a full explanation of the benefits, risks, and dietary/medication restrictions. The starting dose is usually 15 mg daily, and this is slowly increased to 45–60 mg a day, and in some cases up to 90 mg a day. The exact amounts vary slightly from one type of MAOI to the next, and detailed instructions are necessary with each. A commonly used drug of this class in the treatment of panic disorder is phenelzine (Nardil).

Common foods and drinks that should be avoided by patients on MAOI drugs are listed in Table 6.

Table 6 Dietary restrictions for patients taking MAOI drugs

Common foods to be avoided

Beer
Broad bean pods
Cheese*
Dry sausage
Foods containing cheese (such as pizza)
Liver
Meat extracts
Over-ripe bananas
Red wine
Smoked or pickled fish, especially herring
Sour cream
Yeast extracts
Yogurt

---

* except cottage cheese and cream cheese in moderate quantities.
Note: This is not an exhaustive list.

Some members of a class of drugs that are known to reduce anxiety, the benzodiazepines, have also been shown to reduce panic frequency. Their effects can be relatively quick. The drug alprazolam (Xanax), which is a high-potency benzodiazepine, has been intensively investigated and is often prescribed for panic disorder. However, withdrawal can be difficult with benzodiazepines, and it is therefore desirable to taper off the dosage slowly. The relapse rate after terminating the medication is high, in some reports up to 90%.

The common side-effects include sleepiness, light-headedness, and slowing down of physical and mental activity. Less frequent effects include fatigue, slurred speech, and forgetfulness. There are risks of dependence with benzodiazepines, and for this reason they are not prescribed for patients who have abused alcohol or drugs. The exact dose varies between medications, but alprazolam is generally started at a low dose of 0.5 mg, three times daily, increasing up to 6 mg daily. In some cases a dose of 10 mg is needed. The increase in the dosage is done in small steps, and abrupt withdrawal of the medication is avoided.

In summary, imipramine is the most widely used drug for panic disorder. If imipramine is poorly tolerated or insufficient, other anti-depressants from the same group (tricyclics) are used. If these are not satisfactory, a selected benzodiazepine such as alprazolam may be prescribed, with due attention paid to the potential problems of withdrawal effects or relapse. The MAOI anti-depressants offer a third possibility, and are used with particular care because of the risks and prohibitions.

Of course, the decision about what medication to use and at what dosage, always depends on the doctor's assessment of the individual patient, and it is common for patients to be prescribed different medication at different times. In every case, both the progress and the side-effects are carefully monitored, and adjustments are made as necessary. The comments above are intended to give only a broad and general picture.

Psychological treatment

Prior to the recognition of panic disorder as a distinct condition, most people who suffered from panics and who also feared and avoided such things as public transport, enclosed places, and driving were given the diagnosis of agoraphobia. The main psychological treatment for agoraphobia was systematic desensitization to the feared places, and/or planned exercises that consisted of entering the feared places for increasingly long periods. In both of these treatments the affected person was gradually and systematically exposed to the objects of their fears; in the classical version, systematic desensitization, the exposures took places in imagined rehearsals during relaxation, and in the second treatment, the exposures took place in the real situations. Both methods were examples of 'behaviour therapy'.

Roughly 10 years ago, an important new component was added to behaviour therapy techniques. Therapists began to focus attention on eliciting the patient's cognitions about their fears (such as their thoughts, beliefs, ideas, and attitudes) and then helping to modify those cognitions that are harmful or wrong. This expansion of behaviour therapy is appropriately labelled cognitive–behaviour therapy, and it has become the mainstay of psychological treatment for panic disorder. Before describing the details of these treatments, some background information may be helpful.

Behaviour therapy, also called behaviour modification or behavioural psychotherapy, refers to the use of learning theory in the treatment of psychological disorders. Learning theory is the body of knowledge and ideas that psychologists have developed on the basis of hundreds of studies of how changes take place in human and animal behaviour. The use of this knowledge, and techniques based on it, for human psychological disorders was always considered possible, and several people in the early part of this century reported such use. However, it was only in the 1950s that it developed into a formalized treatment approach. This was largely due to the work of the South African psychiatrist Joseph Wolpe, who later practised in Temple University, Philadelphia. The work of Hans Eysenck in London contributed greatly to the development and acceptance of behaviour therapy as a major approach to certain psychological problems. This approach views many behavioural problems as learned, as cases of faulty or 'maladaptive' learning, or as cases of failure to learn. It should be possible to correct the disorder by applying the principles of learning: the faulty learning can be undone, and new learning can be promoted. Therefore, behaviour therapy concentrates on the problem behaviour itself rather than an assumed root cause. This is in contrast to the psychoanalytic approach of Freud and his followers who saw behavioural problems as symptoms of a deeper, unconscious problem. Behaviour therapists concentrate more on the problem as it is now, and what factors are currently associated with it, rather than its past history. Of course, therapists need to know from the patient when the problem started, how it developed, and so on, but the main focus is on the problem as it is now, and the therapist's efforts are geared towards modifying this problem.

The efficacy of behaviour therapy for a range of psychological disorders is well established. For many of these, it is now considered by many clinicians to be the treatment of choice. The early criticism that if a problem is treated directly by behaviour therapy, without going into its 'unconscious roots', it will later lead to other symptoms, has been shown to be unfounded. There is no evidence that such symptom substitution takes place. Cognitive–behaviour therapy, as mentioned earlier, is the result of expanding the scope of behaviour therapy to include aspects of what is known as cognitive therapy. Cognitive therapists focus their treatment on the patient's cognitions and on helping them to modify them. The most impressive work by cognitive therapists so far has been in the treatment of depression. Depressed patients often have very negative thoughts such as 'I am a worthless person', 'There is no point in my life', and so on. Attempts are made to modify these using a variety of techniques, including challenging the maladaptive thoughts, showing evidence to the contrary, and setting up situations in which they are disconfirmed. This last element is, of course, a behavioural one.

The value of cognitive–behaviour therapy was first established in depression, and these principles and techniques are now being used for other disorders as well, notably panic disorder.

Details of psychological treatment

In the following paragraphs, a fairly detailed account of the psychological therapy for panic disorder is given.

Exposure exercises

The exercises that were developed for the treatment of agoraphobia retain their value in the treatment of panic disorder, particularly if the patient's activities and travel have become restricted. In the original exposure method (systematic desensitization), the patient was given a course of relaxation training and then asked to imagine the fearful situations/activities while in a state of deep relaxation. The fearful images are ranked from least to most disturbing, and presented in a graded and gradual manner starting with the least fearful. The ranking is commonly done on the basis of the subjective fear ratings given by the patient, usually on a 0–100 scale (see Chapter 8, p. 59). With repeated practice the images become less and less fearful, and the patient is then urged to facilitate the transfer of these increasing fearless reactions from imagination into the real situation.

For example, while relaxing, the patient who is afraid of travelling by bus might start by imagining riding in a bus for one stop. After several repetitions the fear reaction will decline. After overcoming an item in the list, the patient then tackles the next most fearful item. When the patient's fears have reduced and they are ready, they will be encouraged to actually take a short bus ride. The whole process is gradual, methodical, and progressive—and cushioned by relaxation.

Unfortunately, systematic desensitization can be a lengthy process, and the transfer from fearless imagination to fearless performance is by no means assured. In many instances the transfer is incomplete or simply fails to occur.

For reasons of efficiency and superior therapeutic results, the imaginal exposure technique was largely replaced by exposure exercises that take place in the real situations, so-called *in vivo* exposures. As in systematic desensitization, a list of fearful situations is compiled, ranging from the least to the most frightening, which is then used in planing the exposure exercises, which take place daily if possible, or as frequently as is practical. The hierarchy is used flexibly, depending on circumstances, but the plan is to move progressively from the least to the most frightening situation.

The following is a simplified example of a fear hierarchy:

(1) walking to the gate of a nearby park, accompanied by a trusted adult;

(2) walking 100 yards into the park, accompanied;

(3) staying in the park for 10 minutes, accompanied;

(4) walking to the gate of the park, alone;

(5) walking into the park, alone.

The patient is required to keep a complete diary that includes each exercise and the degree of anxiety present before, during, and after the exercise, plus the time and distances, and any panicky feelings. An example of a record sheet from such a diary is given in Figure 7 (see p.76).

To continue the example:

Item 1, walking to nearby park, accompanied, 30 minutes, April 12, a.m.
  Anxiety before = 80/100
  Anxiety during = 70/100
  Anxiety after = 55/100

Item 1, repeat, 30 minutes, April 13, a.m.
  Anxiety before = 60/100
  Anxiety during = 50/100
  Anxiety after = 30/100

Item 2, walking 100 yards into park, accompanied, 45 minutes, April 14, a.m.
  Anxiety before = 65/100
  Anxiety during = 30/100
  Anxiety after = 20/100

In most instances the first few exposure exercises are carried out while accompanied by a therapist or aide. As the patient's fear begins to subside with repeated exercises, the therapist gradually distances him/herself in a planned manner, and finally fades out of the picture altogether.

As in systematic desensitization, relaxation may be used as a technique for suppressing fear. Typically, patients are trained to relax themselves, and then encouraged to induce feelings of relaxation before and during exposure exercises, and whenever they begin to feel high levels of anxiety.

Cognitive therapy of panic

Cognitive therapy is based on the idea that panics are caused by catastrophic misinterpretations of certain bodily sensations (see Chapter 5). Therefore, in order to eliminate panics, it is necessary to modify the catastrophic misinterpretations in a more realistic and accurate direction, and/or reduce the severity and frequency with which the person experiences the bodily sensations. This has several benefits. The introduction or restoration of safer and more realistic interpretations of these sensations should ensure that few or no panics are experienced. Furthermore, a reduction in the severity and frequency of the bodily sensations should reduce the opportunities for making catastrophic misinterpretations. Finally, therapy usually includes steps to combat any maladaptive avoidance behaviour that might have emerged as a consequence of the episodes of panic.

Identification. In order to modify the maladaptive cognitions it is necessary first to identify them. After obtaining a full description of the type and frequency of panic episodes which the person has experienced, the next step is to obtain a detailed description of a few recent episodes of panic, and as full an account of the first episode of panic as it is possible to regain.

These descriptions include the circumstances in which the panic took place, the bodily reactions that were experienced, the behaviour associated with the panic, and most importantly, the thoughts which the person had immediately before and during the episode of panic. Usually, it is possible to detect the occurrence of significant bodily sensations and associated thoughts, and also to obtain an inkling of whether or not the same thoughts are repeatedly involved in the episodes.

For example, a patient whose episodes of panic appeared to occur without rhyme or reason, and in unexpected places at unexpected times, turned out to have a highly specific link between a particular bodily sensation and the experience of panic. After a close analysis that occupied four sessions and some behavioural tests, it emerged that she had experienced an inner ear infection that seriously interfered with her balance, which cleared up after taking a course of antibiotic medication. A week later, when she was out in a shopping mall with her three young children, she had a recurrence of dizziness and fell to the ground. With assistance, she was able gradually to recall the thoughts that she had experienced at the time of this incident. Initially she felt that she was fainting and that there was something wrong with her brain; her anxieties turned immediately to the safety of her three children. She was frightened that if she lost consciousness or worse, her children would be left unprotected and at risk.

In the course of the next six months she experienced eight more episodes of panic, at seemingly unconnected and inexplicable times and places, but they appeared to have a common element of feelings of dizziness or a threat of fainting, losing consciousness, or even dying. Her episodes of panic appeared to be triggered by feelings of dizziness, sometimes even very slight feelings of which she was not fully aware; in addition, she had rapidly become sensitized to the shopping mall in which the first incident occurred, and to similar situations. She began to feel apprehensive anxiety whenever she had to re-enter the original shopping mall or others like it, which then contributed to the feeling of dizziness itself, establishing a vicious circle.

Expectations of panic. After collecting from the patient detailed descriptions of the original episode and recent panics, information is gathered about the circumstances in which attacks are most likely to occur, and when they are likely to be severe. A common factor in determining the likelihood of a panic and its severity is the presence of a trusted adult. The reasoning behind these variations in expectations of panic usually follows this pattern: 'If the pounding of my heart is an indication that I might be on the verge of a heart attack, then I am in greatest danger when alone at some distance from medical services.

If, however, I am accompanied by a trusted adult, or if I am near to emergency medical services, the dangers are less serious. Travelling alone to an inaccessible part of the country, especially on my own, is far too risky.'

Information is also collected about the actions or situations that might prevent an episode of panic or that would make it less severe or troubling. In addition to the presence of a trusted adult and medical services, the availability of a trusted medication may dampen down or may even prevent an episode of panic. The availability of a thoroughly reliable motor vehicle helps, as does the knowledge that one's family doctor is in town and easily accessible. It is not uncommon for patients to increase their medications whenever their doctor is out of town.

Patients often have in-situation safety behaviour which they regularly use, and details of these are also sought. This behaviour includes, for example, tensing one's legs, holding on to solid objects like tables and railings, and sitting down if there is a fear of fainting.

Time is taken to learn about the attitudes and behaviour of other people towards the episodes of panic, and especially, of course, the attitude and behaviour of close family members, and employers and colleagues. It is important also to attempt to understand the patient's beliefs about the nature of the problem and what caused it.

As will be described in the section on assessment (Chapter 8), it often is extremely useful and indeed necessary to link the information which is collected during the clinical interview to a series of behavioural experiments. These enable the sufferer and the therapist to confirm or disconfirm whatever ideas have emerged about the underlying beliefs that are propelling the panic problem, and they frequently provide fresh information about the cognitions and other aspects of the panic episodes.

Treatment begins.   Once the assessment has been completed, and some likely candidates for the source of the catastrophic thoughts have been identified, the actual treatment process begins. The therapist gives the patient a good deal of information about the nature of anxiety, episodes of panic, and the role of cognitions in causing the emotional reactions. Some patients rapidly recognize the extent to which their own experiences and thoughts fit in with this information, and find it very reassuring that their experiences are familiar, well-described, reasonably well understood, common to many people, and responsive to treatment. The patient can change from a frightened and bewildered sufferer, tormented by a possibly sinister disorder, into a person who recognizes that they simply have a problem with controlling anxiety. Patients also welcome a form of treatment in which they take an active part with the therapist in searching for understanding and explanation, not only of their present difficulties, but of the events which led up to them. The transition from a passive sufferer, who has undergone a frightening and poorly understood series of unpredictable events, into an active searcher after the nature and causes of the problem, and how to overcome them, is in almost all cases an extremely welcome experience.

It is likely that the introductory educational part of treatment plays a major part in reassuring the patient and providing the basis on which the core of the treatment is based.

Linkages. Certain links between sensations and catastrophic thoughts are particularly common. These include: the connection between the sensation of a pounding heart and the fear of an imminent heart attack; shortness of breath and fear that one will suffocate and die; the sensation of feeling faint and the thought of passing out or dying; and unusual sensations in the head, or unusual perceptions, and the fear that one is going mad.

These links can be extremely important, and they are not always obvious. Frequently patients are surprised when they learn about the strength and frequency with which they make these connections between particular sensations and specific frightening thoughts of catastrophe. Furthermore, these links between sensations and catastrophic cognitions often are associated with vivid and frightening images, as the following case histories illustrate.

● ●

A young man complained of panic attacks accompanied by shortness of breath and his legs feeling weak. He was terrified that he would collapse and die when this happened. He had a vivid visual image, which came to him at the time, of himself lying on the ground, gasping for breath, looking hideous. Just as he began to feel the shortness of breath, the image always came. This added to his fear and distress.

A 35-year-old female lecturer complained of panic attacks of over a year's duration, which began when her mother was seriously ill. The first thing

*that happened in her panics was feeling faint. As soon as she felt like
this, she felt terrified that she would die. She had a sharp image of her
mother in a coffin, as indeed she had seen her after she died, and another
identical coffin, in which she could see her own 'corpse'. The image was
vivid and distinct, and came instantly, convincing her that she was about
to drop dead.*

• •

Changing cognitions.   Once the patient and therapist are reasonably
sure that they have identified important links, a number of techniques
are introduced that will help the person to gain more appropriate and
safer interpretations of events.

These techniques include: the search for alternative explanations;
considering how other people would interpret the situation; the
inclusion of important facts that have been omitted, or the deletion
of misleading facts that are being unnecessarily included; and trying to
estimate the true probability that the catastrophic event will actually
take place.

'What evidence do I have for this thought?' 'Is there any alternative
way of looking at the situation?' 'Is there any alternative explanation?'
These questions, which are among the most commonly used, are
illustrated in the transcript below, which also highlights the value
of providing information about anxiety. This transcript, from a case
extract described by Dr David Clark, provides a particularly good
example of the search for an alternative explanation.

Patient	'In the middle of a panic attack, I usually think I am going to faint or collapse.'
Therapist	'How much do you believe that sitting here right now, and how much would you believe it if you had the sensations you get in an attack?'
Patient	'50% now and 90% in an attack.'
Therapist	'OK, let's look at the evidence you have for this thought. Have you ever fainted in an attack?'
Patient	'No.'
Therapist	'What is it then that makes you think you might faint?'

Patient   'I feel faint and the feeling can be very strong.'

Therapist   'So, to summarize, your evidence that you are going to faint is the fact that you feel faint?'

Patient   'Yes.'

Therapist   'How can you then account for the fact that you have felt faint many hundreds of times and have not yet fainted?'

Patient   'So far, the attacks have always stopped just in time or I have managed to hold onto something to stop myself from collapsing.'

Therapist   'Right, so one explanation of the fact that you have frequently felt faint, and the thought that you will faint, but have not actually fainted, is that you have always done something to save yourself just in time. However, an alternative explanation is that the feeling of faintness that you get in a panic attack will never lead to you collapsing, even if you don't control it.'

Patient   'Yes, I suppose so.'

Therapist   'In order to decide which of these two possibilities is correct, we need to know what has to happen to your body for you to actually faint. Do you know?'

Patient   'No.'

Therapist   'Your blood pressure needs to drop. Do you know what happens to your blood pressure during a panic attack?'

Patient   'Well, my pulse is racing. I guess my blood pressure must be up.'

Therapist   'That's right. In anxiety, heart rate and blood pressure tend to go together. So, you are actually *less* likely to faint when you are anxious then when you are not.'

Patient   'That's very interesting and helpful to know. However, if it's true, why do I feel so faint?'

Therapist   'Your feeling of faintness is a sign that your body is reacting in a normal way to the perception of danger. Most of the bodily reactions you are experiencing when anxious were probably designed to deal with the threats experienced by primitive man, such as being approached by a hungry tiger. What would be the best thing to do in that situation?'

Patient   'Run away as fast as you can.'

Therapist 'That's right. And in order to help you run, you need the maximum amount of energy in your muscles. This is achieved by sending more of your blood to your muscles and relatively less to the brain. This means that there is a small drop in oxygen to the brain and this is why you *feel* faint. However, this feeling is misleading in the sense that it doesn't mean you will actually faint because your overall blood pressure is up, not down.'

Patient   'That's very clear. So next time I feel faint, I can check out whether I am going to faint by taking my pulse. If it is normal, or quicker than normal, I know I won't faint.'

Therapist 'That's right. Now, on the basis of what we've discussed so far, how much do you believe you might faint in a panic attack?'

Patient   'Less, say 10%.'

Therapist 'And if you were experiencing the sensation?'

Patient   'Maybe 25%.'

(This case excerpt is from Clark (1989). Reproduced with permission.)

The underlying fear of going insane is illustrated in the following case:

• •

Mr S., a 35-year-old sales manager, complained of repeated episodes of panic that were distressing and also interfering with his ability to make business calls. On examination it appeared that most of the episodes of panic, and those which were near-panics, took place shortly before or at the beginning of a business call. The patient had been extremely shy as a child and had, with difficulty, gained sufficient confidence to enter business sales. It turned out that there were certain kinds of customers or settings in which he felt a surge of social anxiety, and during these periods he felt extremely dizzy and felt that he was babbling incoherently. He then became extremely frightened and at times had full-blown episodes of panic. Analysis revealed that he was interpreting those periods of dizziness, and what he took to be incoherent speech, as signs that he might be having a nervous breakdown, and possibly going insane. His idea of insanity, which was incorrect, had been constructed without his realizing it, on the basis of some frightening visits which he made as an adolescent to see an elderly uncle who was a long-term resident in a psychiatric hospital. The uncle suffered from chronic schizophrenia and was unresponsive for most of the time, other than making requests for cigarettes, prefaced and followed by incoherent mumbling.

When, as an adult salesman, he became socially anxious and felt that he was not speaking clearly, the patient automatically interpreted this as an early sign of impending mental illness. He then had some harrowing images of himself, disabled and deteriorated, as he had seen his uncle. With the aid of the therapist, Mr S. compiled a list of the main signs of mental illness, including schizophrenia, and in another column he listed his own experiences and 'symptoms'. In the construction of this list of comparisons between the symptoms of schizophrenia and his own experiences, it became apparent that the differences were overwhelming, and gradually he lost his fear of developing schizophrenia as his uncle had done. He had no further panics, but continued to feel uneasy in awkward social situations.

● ●

Behavioural experiments The analysis and discussion of a patient's past experiences and interpretations of events is a necessary step in identifying the cognitive origin of panic. However, the mere identification of the thoughts and attitudes may not be sufficient. Certainly, the balancing of evidence for and against a particular thought, such as the possibility of having a heart attack, may be too abstract, too removed from the actual situation to be of sufficient help. Moreover, most patients distinguish between the thoughts they have in the calm safety of the clinic, and the thoughts they have during a panic episode. In these instances the use of so-called behavioural experiments can be extremely helpful. In addition to confirming or disconfirming the value of different sorts of evidence, they can be used to collect fresh information. And it has to be said that in many instances, it is episodes of personal experience that are most effective in bringing about changes in beliefs; sometimes the patient can achieve in one successful behavioural exercise far more than hours of discussion and analysis will yield.

To take a case example, a 25-year-old man complained of repeated episodes of panic. The episodes were severe and tended mostly to occur when he engaged in rigorous physical exercise. As a result, he had given up weight-lifting and jogging, even though he valued the exercise and regretted the decline in his physical condition that ensued when he gave up these activities. Analysis suggested that the panic episodes generally were brought on by a strong sensation of a pounding heart and oppression in the chest, which he often experienced after or during a strenuous session of weight-lifting (one wonders whether weight-lifting is ever not strenuous). In certain vulnerable moods he automatically interpreted the chest sensations and pounding heart as signs that he was about to have a heart attack, and naturally felt extremely frightened. He reported that the episodes of panic which took place in these circumstances tended to last 15–20 minutes. In the course of a discussion about the possible interpretations of these physical sensations, the patient and therapist compiled a list of evidence supporting an interpretation that he was about to have a heart attack, versus a list of information suggesting instead that the symptoms were due to an anxious misinterpretation of the chest and heart sensations. It turned out that the patient was well aware that people who have heart conditions often experience tightness of the chest and shortness of breath as a result of vigorous exercising, but that sufferers quickly gain some relief and composure by sitting down and resting. In contrast, the same sensations that result from anxiety do not respond to the simple expedient of sitting down and resting. From his own experience, he knew that these episodes of panic, once started, tended to last from 15–20 minutes—even while resting.

In order to test these alternative interpretations, and also to give him the experience of 'surviving' a period of vigorous exercise and subsequent heart and chest sensations, a specific behavioural test was formulated. The aim was to check the effects of a period of physical rest on the patient's feelings of panic and the associated bodily sensations of chest tension and rapid heartbeat. It was agreed in advance that if the patient's unpleasant chest and heart sensations continued unchanged for up to 20 minutes after taking a rest from exercise, this result would be most consistent with the idea that the sensations were symptoms of anxiety, rather than the early signs of a heart attack. On the other hand, if they lasted for less than 20 minutes after resting, anxiety was unlikely to be the cause.

The behavioural test was duly carried out on two separate occasions. The first attempt to induce panicky feelings during vigorous physical exercise that included weight-lifting proved to be unsuccessful. The patient had become aware that he was sweating and that his heart had increased its rate, but there were no alarming physical sensations, and it was therefore impossible to test the effects of the pre-arranged rest period. On the second attempt, however, about 20 minutes into the vigorous exercising he began to be alarmed by feelings of pressure in his chest and by a racing heart. As on a number of previous episodes, he began to feel panicky, and to think that he might be in the early stages of a heart attack. Fortunately, he was nevertheless able to carry out the test as planned. He sat down in a comfortable chair for 30 minutes, and found that the uncomfortable sensations and the panicky feeling persisted unchanged for 18 minutes before entering a slow decline. Even though he was resting, the cardiac sensations persisted.

When the results of the two tests were discussed, the patient concluded that they were more consistent with the interpretation that he was experiencing anxiety rather than an imminent heart attack. The behavioural tests also gave rise to a memory that he felt was relevant. Apparently he had heard about a year ago that an elderly uncle of one of his acquaintances had had a serious heart attack while exercising at a local gymnasium. Furthermore, he was able to remember that, during a number of panic episodes associated with exercising, he had definitely had thoughts and images of the old man suddenly being struck down by a heart attack.

Patients whose panicky thoughts incorporate a fear of imminent medical catastrophe, such as a heart attack, readily agree that their panicky feelings decrease when they are distracted. The question is: Can anyone distract themselves from a heart attack, or other catastrophes, such as brain tumours or loss of consciousness? The effects of distraction can provide the basis for valuable experiments on the patients' fears and reactions.

Overcoming avoidance behaviour

As described earlier, the main weapon against excessive avoidance behaviour is the introduction of planned and methodical exposure exercises. To some extent, these exposure exercises also function as behavioural tests in that some of the person's maladaptive cognitions are challenged and disconfirmed during the conduct of the exercises. For example, the idea that one might become dizzy and then faint on a bus can be put to repeated behavioural tests by planned journeys on selected bus routes, usually starting with the easiest journey and the least crowded buses, and then progressively moving towards more difficult bus rides. The patient learns that even if they do experience sensations of faintness, these never progress to the point of losing consciousness. Plainly, if one persistently avoids going on the bus, the belief that the sensations of faintness are a sure sign of an impending loss of consciousness will never the tested, and hence can never be disconfirmed.

An important aspect of exposure exercises involves the patient's habitual safety behaviour in panic-provoking situations. In treatment, the patient is asked not to carry out these in-situation safety behaviours. For example, a patient may hold on to solid objects when he fears he is going to faint. The patient can be encouraged to test his belief that he will faint by moving away from solid objects, which is often an important part of treatment.

Relapse prevention

In order to prevent a relapse from occurring, the closing sessions of treatment become increasingly educational. These closing sessions are widely spaced, and patients are encouraged to take on more and more of the planning and conduct of the treatment so that they can become independent, and gain increasing self-confidence about their ability to deal with and control the problem unassisted. Patients are also given advice about circumstances in which recurrences might occur, such as fresh stresses or conflicts, losses or bereavements, episodes of ill health, the introduction of new catastrophic cognitions, and so forth. Some time is spent in going over how the patient can recognize the signs of a possible return of panic, and what they should do to prevent it from recurring. For example: 'If you notice that you are becoming increasingly sensitive to your heart beat and starting to have frightening ideas or images, restart your daily recordings and try to find what, if anything, is triggering the thoughts and images. Once you have that information, set down the evidence for and against at least two alternative interpretations, and then proceed to test them. If you find yourself starting to avoid situations for reasons of fear, that is the surest sign that you need to enter those situations repeatedly, and remain there for increasing periods of time.'

Patients are also told that if the problem becomes unmanageable, they are welcome to seek further assistance, and reminded that booster or retreatment sessions are generally successful and require comparatively few visits. For many patients, the mere knowledge that the channels remain open is sufficient to provide that degree of security which enables them to manage largely unassisted.

Combined psychological and pharmacological treatment

Some psychiatrists take the approach that panic disorder should be treated with drugs to begin with followed by psychological therapy once some control over the attacks is achieved. There are others who advocate concurrent drug and psychological teatment. A number of attempts have been made to combine psychological treatment and medication in the hope of producing stronger effects. This is a plausible expectation; however, a combination of the two methods does not appear to produce better results. There is some concern about whether or not the tendency to relapse when medication is stopped might also have an adverse effect on the psychological treatment. The available evidence suggests that this can be avoided if the drug is withdrawn slowly and carefully.

In practice, large numbers of patients receive a combination of psychological and pharmacological treatments. There appears to be little reason for concern about the combination, assuming it is sensibly done. Equally, there is so far no compelling evidence that the combination leads to major advantages. In those cases where drug treatment has been used initially with beneficial effect, following this with some treatment using psychological principles is likely to reduce the chances of relapse.

7   *Further aspects of treatment*
●●

Primary care of panic disorders

During the first experience of panic, especially if it occurs unexpectedly (spontaneously), it is common for people to seek medical help. In numerous cases the person goes to, or is transported to, an emergency medical facility, particularly if they feel in danger of having a heart attack. The young woman described on p.1, who experienced chest pains and breathing difficulties, felt that she was having a heart attack, and her husband rushed her to the nearest hospital emergency clinic. After a full examination the doctors reassured her that her heart was entirely normal, and she went home feeling shaken and anxious but relieved. When, a few days later, she had her second panic, she realized that a serious and puzzling health problem had emerged and consulted her family doctor.

In the early stages of the disorder, sufferers from unrecognized panic disorder will do the same as anyone facing a serious, imminent threat to their health—urgently seek medical care. After the first one or two episodes of panic, it becomes clear that the problem cannot be dealt with by visits to the emergency clinic of a hospital. It is common at this stage to visit one's family doctor, who in some cases may deal with the problem. However, if the problem is not resolved at this facility, a referral to a specialist service such as a clinical psychologist or a psychiatrist may follow.

Patients who consult their family doctor after episodes of intense fear accompanied by disturbing bodily sensations and a sense of impending catastrophe may be suffering from one of a variety of problems other than panic disorder. After the doctor successfully rules out the other possibilities, attention is paid to specific episodes and the presence or absence of additional stresses in the two months prior to the first episode.

A diagnosis of panic disorder is made if the patient has had repeated episodes of panic within the past month or two, at least some of which were 'spontaneous' and were followed by prolonged feelings of anxiety and apprehension. The early signs of significant avoidance behaviour is a confirming feature.

If the family doctor does not already have the information, they will assess the presence/absence of previous periods of anxiety, and collect data on recent stressful events or anticipated events, and their possible relation to the panics. Because of the common association of panic with depression, the assessment will include a search for signs of depression (feelings of helplessness, despair, crying, insomnia, loss of energy/interest). Patients with panic disorder report feeling frightened when they feel short of breath, and/or feel faint, and/or feel shaky, and/or their heart beats rapidly.

If a diagnosis is made of panic disorder, the family doctor is in an excellent position to provide education and reassuring explanations, supplemented if possible by reading materials, and to advise the patient about expected developments and the need to avoid excessive drinking of caffeine or use of other stimulants. The patient will also be encouraged to attempt to maintain their normal daily activities and to 'avoid avoidance'. Depending on the severity and frequency of the panics and anxiety, medication may or may not be prescribed. If the panics and/or anxiety and avoidance persist and are distressing or disabling, specialist treatment may be required.

Hyperventilation (overbreathing)

Disturbed breathing is a typical response to a threatening event (such as an unexplained noise late at night) and, as already noted, feeling short of breath is a common experience during panic episodes. In fact, shortness of breath is one of the most commonly reported and intense panic sensations, the other three being rapid heart beat, sweating, and dizziness. Shortness of breath is also one of the three most intensely felt sensations, along with rapid heart beat and trembling/shaking. People who frequently experience intense feelings of shortness of breath tend to take precautionary measures; they prefer open windows even in cold weather, avoid stale air, and so forth.

A patient who feared a sudden heart attack experienced numerous panics during which his breathing became shallow and rapid, which made him gasp for air and he became particularly sensitive to fresh air. On numerous occasions he fully opened all of the windows of his car when driving in severe winter weather. A school teacher who had a similar problem with overbreathing insisted on keeping open the windows of his classrooms, even during winter. This was not a universally popular move.

Hyperventilation can be a contributing cause of a panic episode, or merely one feature of the episode, albeit an intense and distressing one. Rapid, shallow breathing can produce a number of disturbing bodily reactions such as light-headedness, rapid heart beat, tingling in the fingers and toes, pressure in the chest, and a flushed face. These sensations are unpleasant in themselves, but they can also lead to a full-blown panic.

If the person makes a catastrophic misinterpretation of these unwanted sensations, a panic can occur. Such common misinterpretations include: 'I am light-headed and dizzy, and therefore about to lose consciousness or lose control,' 'My heart is pounding (and that means) I am in danger of straining my heart and dying,' and 'The pressure in my chest is a symptom of an oncoming heart attack'.

Hyperventilation tests

In the assessment phase, patients may be asked to undertake a brief test in order to determine whether or not hyperventilation is playing a part in the episodes of panic. The reason for, and the nature of, the test is explained in order to obtain the patient's informed consent and co-operation. A typical test takes place as follows:

'I would like you to carry out a short, simple test of your breathing. When I ask you to begin, please start breathing shallowly and rapidly, and continue to do so until I ask you to stop at the end of two minutes. If you wish to do so, you can, of course, stop at any time, but do try to continue for the full two minutes if you can.

'Before we begin, please tell me if you are at all anxious at present. Use a 0–100 scale, a sort of thermometer of anxiety in which 0 is completely calm and 100 is terror. You can use any part of the scale, so 20/100 would indicate very slight anxiety, 50/100 moderate anxiety, 80/100 intense fear, and so on. What is your score at present, out of 100?

'Are you aware of any bodily sensations at present?'

(After ensuring that the patient understands the instructions, the therapist begins the test.)

'Now begin overbreathing and try to continue until I tell you that the two minutes are up. Please go ahead.'

(Sometimes it is necessary for the therapist to demonstrate the overbreathing exercise in order to make sure the patient understands what is needed.)

At the end of the test period the patient re-rates his/her anxiety, 0–100, and is also asked to describe any new or persisting bodily sensations. Commonly the test result is positive and the patient recognizes that some of the feelings resemble those that they have experienced during episodes of panic. One patient observed: 'It was very similar to how I feel during a panic, but somehow less real, less frightening.'

The results of the hyperventilation test can be revealing, as in the case of a 42-year-old woman who had repeatedly experienced extremely intense episodes of panic. During the hyperventilation test she initially became very dizzy and light-headed, and those reactions then developed into a major panic. It turned out that the dizziness, light-headedness, and pressure she felt in her head during the overbreathing triggered a thought that she had something wrong in her brain. Further analysis revealed that the underlying, terrifying thought was that she had a cancerous tumour in the brain. Eight years earlier, she had undergone surgery for the successful removal of a cancerous tumour of the breast, but was plagued by fears of a recurrence of the cancer in other parts of her body. (Her mother and a maternal aunt had both died of secondary cancers.) One of the major causes of her panics was the catastrophic misinterpretation of the sensations produced by spontaneous overbreathing, and she subsequently derived relief from a recognition of this connection and a course of breathing retraining.

People who habitually hyperventilate can learn to regulate and control their breathing with little difficulty. With practice, they acquire the ability to impose a slow, steady rhythm on their breathing at will, reducing the tendency to overbreathe. For some, the use of a small paper bag proves helpful. The effects of overbreathing, including the unpleasant associated sensations, sometimes are reversible within minutes of breathing into a paper bag that fits snugly over the nose and mouth.

It is not known for certain why some people habitually overbreathe, but at least two contributing factors have been identified. Firstly, people who have had some respiratory illness or difficulties (such as asthma) seem to be at some risk of overbreathing. Secondly, people who have an intense fear of suffocation are also inclined to overbreathe, perhaps in compensation for their worries about not getting sufficient air into their lungs.

In many cases there is a connection between panic disorder and the fear of suffocation, which can provide the basis for episodes of panic: any threat to one's air supply, whether a true threat or a catastrophic misinterpretation of events, can provoke a panic. Hence, people who strongly fear suffocation are at an increased risk for panic when they find themselves in a small, enclosed space. It is just the setting in which a panic can occur. Indeed, in laboratory research one of the most reliable ways of provoking mild panics is by asking people to remain for a few minutes in a small enclosure such as a kiosk or chamber.

Hyperventilation tests: a caution

It is important to stress that hyperventilation tests should not be attempted in certain medical conditions. These include: epilepsy, hypertension, hypotension, asthma and other respiratory diseases, and cardiovascular illness. They should not be performed during pregnancy.

Breathing retraining

Breathing retraining, which is often incorporated into a general course of relaxation training, is especially useful in the treatment of panic disorder, particularly if the patient is prone to hyperventilate. The aim of the training is to teach the person to adopt a slow, paced rate of breathing, at will, and to use the method whenever they begin to overbreathe.

Patients are taught to breathe smoothly and slowly, reducing the rate from 16 to 20 breaths per minute to roughly 8 breaths per minute. After observing the rate and pattern of the patient's breathing, the therapist begins to pace it.

'Now that you are in a comfortable, relaxed position, please concentrate on your breathing. Take a deep breath in through your nose ... fill your lungs ... Good, now hold that for one second ... and now release all the air. Expel it all, and release any tension in your body as you expel the air.

'Now, once again fill your lungs ... take a slow deep breath ... hold it ... Now release, let it all go.

'Breathe in ... hold it ... release it.'

After a few minutes of slow, paced breathing the therapist encourages the patient to repeat the instructions to themselves: 'Now I would like you to repeat to yourself the breathing instructions. Keep to a regular, rhythmic pattern. Breathe in ... hold it ... breathe out ... breathe in ... breathe out.

'From now on, try to control your own breathing in this way, whenever the need arises.'

Patients learn the method easily and quickly, and commonly find that it relieves tension and adds to a general feeling of relaxation. They are encouraged to use slow, paced breathing in their everyday activities, especially if they start overbreathing and/or feeling the bodily sensations (such as numbness) that are part of their pattern of panics. They are also encouraged to think of paced, slow breathing as a means of controlling their otherwise unruly, troubling reactions.

Other methods of breathing training have also been recommended by therapists. One such method is increasing the movement of the diaphragm, especially during inhalation.

8 *Assessment and evaluation*

Aims of assessment

Assessment is carried out to determine the nature of the problem, and to make a diagnosis. Later, in the course of treatment, assessments are used to evaluate progress. The criteria used in the diagnosis of panic disorder were described in Chapter 1, and seldom present a major problem. The criteria are set out clearly and the necessary information can be collected without difficulty: the occurrence of repeated episodes of intense fear of sudden onset, some of which are unexpected and which peak within minutes, accompanied by a number of bodily sensations. Those diagnostic problems that do arise generally concern the coexistence of other disorders, and the relationship between these and the panic disorder itself.

Once the diagnosis is established, further and more detailed assessments are undertaken, the main purpose of which is to gain information for devising a treatment programme. The selection of a pharmacological treatment will be influenced by the presence or absence of problems additional to the panic disorder for example, physical illnesses, and take into account the patient's reactions to previous medications, if any. Much of the same information collected to make a decision about medication, and to evaluate the effects of such medication, is common to the assessment procedures that are carried out in planning psychological treatment.

Methods of assessment

Interview

The main method of assessment is the clinical interview, which may take up to three hours to complete and is sometimes spread over more than one session. The patient is asked for full details of the problem, including the way in which it affects their work, social life, and relationships. Questions will be asked about how and when it all started and what the course of the disorder has been, including fluctuations in severity, relation to stressful events, and so on. Most clinicians follow one of the standardized procedures for carrying out such interviews.

It is particularly important for purposes of the original diagnosis and for the later evaluation to have a full and clear description of the episodes of panic. The patient is asked to describe the first, and the most recent panics in considerable detail. Some of the key details are reflected in the following questions: Where did it happen? Were you aware of any bodily sensations? What were they? How intense was the fear? What did you think was happening to you? What action did you take, if any? Did it come on you suddenly? How long did it last? Do you have any ideas about what caused it?

An attempt is then made to find out whether the early and recent episodes are similar, or whether they have changed, and it is also important to gain some idea as to whether the episodes being described are typical or unusual. Next, attention is turned to the immediate consequences of the episode of panic: What further action did you take? How did you feel at the end of the episode? What happened on the following and subsequent days? What did you think was happening to you?

Information is then collected about the longer term consequences of the episodes of panic, with particular attention to what avoidance behaviour, if any, has been generated by the episodes of panic.

During the interview, the patient is asked about factors or activities that may prevent or dampen an episode of panic, and what factors appear to precipitate or intensify the episodes of panic.

It is particularly important to get a very clear idea of the person's understanding of the nature and cause of the episodes of panic. The therapist will ask several questions in an attempt to elucidate this.

During the interview, information will also be collected about the personal and family history of the patient. Particular attention must be paid to collecting information about the person's health, and whether any past illnesses feature in the thoughts that are associated with the panics (such as a history of respiratory illnesses, a fear of suffocation during panic). The health history of members of the family, and where relevant, of close friends should be noted. In many instances the person's interpretation of what is happening during the episode of panic is coloured by their knowledge of the illnesses of relatives or friends.

Given the close and common association between panic disorder and depression, the therapist will ask several questions to find out if the person is currently suffering from a significant depression, or has done so in the past, focusing on the two main features of clinical depression: one pertaining to feelings of subjective sadness, helplessness, and worthlessness; and a second feature concerning changes in bodily functions such as insomnia, loss of appetite, loss of sexual drive, and loss of energy.

Often assessment interviews are tape recorded, always with the patient's agreement. Transcripts of the interviews are a valuable record, and enable the therapist to monitor how changes take place over time. For example, it is useful to examine how the patient's understanding of the nature and causes of panic attacks has changed after, say, ten sessions of therapy.

Interviewing others

In many cases it is useful to interview a family member or friend as part of the assessment. Some aspects of the patient's problems may be more clearly described by a family member than by the patient; for example, the problems and stresses caused by the patient's demands and avoidance behaviour may be minimized in the patient's own account. The full extent of the patient's avoidance behaviour may not become apparent until the information is completed by an other person. Most therapists will want to interview a key informant as an essential part of the assessment.

Behavioural tests and direct observation

Sometimes a therapist may carry out one or more behavioural tests with a patient, most commonly to get some idea of the person's range of mobility, and the probability of an episode being provoked in particular settings. The patient's reactions during these test excursions often will provide important information, for example: How long can the patient stay in a crowded supermarket without feeling the urge to escape? What physical sensations are reported while they are there? And, what thoughts are reported as going through their mind? These 'real-life' assessments are relatively easy to set up, and many clinicians include them in their assessment routine.

Subjective ratings

The therapist is also likely to ask the patient to give subjective ratings of fear. Examples were given in Chapter 6 of hierarchies of feared situations used in behavioural therapy. These hierarchies, or lists of events in order of difficulty, are usually constructed on the basis of the patient's ratings of anxiety. The most commonly used rating scale is 0–100, where 0 means no fear at all, and 100 means absolute terror. Patients find this type of scale easy to use. In the assessment of panic disorder, the clinician may ask the patient to give such ratings for fear, urge to flee, likelihood of a severe panic, strength of various beliefs (such as the strength of the belief that the panic attack signifies serious heart disease), and so on. These ratings are also illustrated in the excerpt from Dr David Clark's interview with a patient given on pp.42–44.

Physiological tests

The direct observation of a person during a test walk or other excursion can be supplemented by the collection of physiological information, most often a recording of the person's heart rate. During most but not all episodes of panic, the patient's heart rate increases by anything from 3 to 25 beats per minute. When this happens, it is useful to know whether the increase in heart rate precedes or follows the person's feelings of fear and the accompanying thoughts. Physiological recording is not routinely done in most clinics, but some clinicians do include this in their assessment procedure.

Record keeping

It is common for the therapist to ask the patient to keep a daily record of the occurrence of anxiety and/or panic for a week or two prior to starting the active therapy, as a means of establishing a baseline against which to measure later progress. The most common record is a simple weekly diary in which the person records for each day the degree of anxiety that they feel, and the occurrence or non-occurrence of episodes of panic. The panic episodes are described briefly in a separate record with a note of the intensity and duration of the episode and the accompanying sensations and thoughts. An example of a diary is given in Figure 3, and a record of panic episodes is shown in Figure 4. As can be seen, the record focuses on specific problems and these are recorded.

A simply structured weekly diary is easier to use and more meaningful to analyse than unstructured, haphazard accounts. The same applies to the record of panics. These records provide a measure of progress as well as keeping the patient and the therapist informed of any changes in the nature or circumstances of the episodes of panic. The information

Week Commencing:

Day	Highest anxiety (0–100)	Number of panics (if any)
Monday		
Tuesday		
Wednesday		
Thursday		
Friday		
Saturday		
Sunday		

Figure 3   A blank example of a weekly diary.

gathered in the diary and the panic record often helps to clarify the causes, events, or activities that have been contributing to the panics.

Examples of a completed diary and a completed record of panics are given in Figures 5 and 6 respectively.

Self-rated questionnaires

Standard questionnaires are also used for assessment. Indeed, many therapists use them as a routine part of the assessment procedure. They have the advantage of covering a range of difficulties and facilitating the collection of a good deal of information rapidly. They also yield a numerical summary score that can be used in a screening procedure and to get a broad view of progress. These questionnaires, however, are no substitute for interviews, but are used to supplement the information collected during the interview.

The most commonly used instrument with panic disorder patients is the Mobility Inventory, which was briefly mentioned in an earlier chapter (see p.20). It is reproduced in Appendix 1. It consists of 26 items and yields an overall score, plus details about the activities which cause particular problems for the patient in question. A second questionnaire commonly used is the Cognitions Questionnaire, the purpose of which is to obtain some introductory information about the types of frightening thoughts the person may be experiencing.

Date:

Time:

Place:

Alone or accompanied:

If accompanied, by whom:

Activity at the time:

Duration:

Expected or unexpected:

Maximum anxiety felt (0–100):

Physical sensations:

Thoughts:

Outcome — what happened in the end?

Figure 4   A blank example of a record of panic attacks.

Week Commencing: 3 October

Day	Highest anxiety (0–100)	Number of panics (if any)
Monday	70	1
Tuesday	40	0
Wednesday	45	0
Thursday	70	0
Friday	35	0
Saturday	85	1
Sunday	25	0

Figure 5   A completed example of a weekly diary.

Many of the items of this questionnaire were cited in an earlier chapter (see Table 2, p. 8). The patient rates the items to indicate the frequency with which each thought occurred when they were anxious. The ratings are from 0 (thought never occurs) to 5 (thought always occurs). The full questionnaire is given in Appendix 2.

As treatment progresses, the instruments can be readministered to track whether the original avoidance behaviour and fearful thoughts persist or are changing.

These two questionnaires are often supplemented by a question-naire which screens for the presence or absence of depression, most commonly the Beck Depression Inventory. This consists of 21 items and yields an overall score which ranges from 0 to 63. The items cover areas such as sadness, sex drive, appetite, energy, sleep, feelings of guilt, feeling ugly, crying, suicidal thoughts, and so on. For each item, a group of four statements is given, and the patient chooses one (or more) of these as reflecting how they have been in the week up to the day of completing the questionnaire. The statements carry a score of 0, 1, 2, or 3. The score of the chosen statement (or the highest one if more than one is chosen) is counted towards the overall score. Scores above 10 are taken as indicating the presence of mild depression, scores above 16 indicating moderate depression, and scores above 25 indicating severe depression. These cut-off points are, of course, not absolute, and are

Date:	8th October
Time:	About 11.30 a.m.
Place:	Post Office
Alone or accompanied:	Alone
If accompanied, by whom:	–
Activity at the time:	Waiting in queue
Duration:	About 2–3 minutes
Expected or unexpected:	Unexpected

Maximum anxiety felt (0–100): 70

Physical sensations:	shortness of breath
	dizziness
	sweating
	feeling weak
	feeling about to fall
Thoughts:	I am going to collapse here.
	I will make a fool of myself.
	What if I die here.

Outcome – what happened in the end?

Held on to the railing and steadied myself.
Then managed to walk out of the building and got
some fresh air. It was okay then. But I did not
go back into the post office

Figure 6   A completed example of a record of panic attacks.

only used as a rough guide. Like the other scales, the Beck Depression Inventory is readministered at various times in the course of treatment to track the persistence or changes in the patient's depression.

The relationships between the scores on these three instruments are as important as the scores on the individual scales themselves. It is particularly important to see what relationship, if any, there is between depression and the episodes of panic, and how these change during the course of treatment.

It must be noted that, while these are the most commonly used in the assessment of panic disorder patients, there are other questionnaires and inventories that are popular with some therapists. Some examples are: the Anxiety Sensitivity Index, the Panic Attacks Symptoms and Cognitions Questionnaire, the Beck Anxiety Inventory, and the Spielberger State-Trait Anxiety Inventory.

Assessment for evaluating therapy

In a systematic therapeutic approach, the patient will be assessed in some or all of the above ways at several points: before treatment begins, after a period of therapy, at the end of therapy, and at follow-up usually 6 and 12 months later. In this way the patient's progress can be measured formally and methodically. The numerical scores in particular help to highlight the changes in the patient's feelings and behaviour. For example, assuming that therapy has been successful, a patient whose score on the Mobility Inventory was in the clinical range prior to treatment will have fallen to well within the normal range – for example, from 75 to 40. Similarly, a person who started treatment with a significantly high Beck Depression Inventory score of 30, may have a score of less than 10 by the end of treatment indicating an absence of depression. Needless to say, even more important in evaluating the outcome of treatment are the frequency of panic episodes the patient experiences and their ratings of fear. This information will come from the patient's own record-keeping and from interviews.

9 *Obstacles and complications*

· ·

While major progress has been made in developing successful treatments for panic disorder, in practice there are several obstacles and complications.

Drug treatment

The main obstacles to pharmacological treatment are cost, negative attitudes to medication, unpleasant side effects, and restrictions on diet.

As it is often necessary to take medication for long periods, the cost—to the patient or family when the treatment is privately obtained, and to the clinic or hospital when the treatment is provided by the health service—can be a prohibitive factor. Negative attitudes to medication are not uncommon, and may be insuperable for those panic disorder patients who are frightened of any sensations that make them feel they are losing control. For these patients psychological treatment is more appropriate.

There are, as noted earlier, several side-effects of the drugs used to treat panics (see pp. 31–33), and if severe or intrusive these will cause the patient to discontinue medication. Alternative drugs or lower doses may overcome this obstacle. It is highly desirable to prepare patients for possible side-effects and how they might be overcome, and the provision of written material about the medication is recommended. The provision of written and oral information about dietary or other restrictions, and possibly adverse reactions with other drugs, is always important. This is particularly so in the case of MAOI drugs.

The complications of drug treatment include interactions with other medications, and the possibility of relapse when the drugs are withdrawn. Relapses are particularly common with some benzodiazepine drugs, such as alprazolam, although this can sometimes be anticipated and modified by a gradual, tapered withdrawal over a period of up to three months.

Psychological treatment

The obstacles to psychological treatment are cost, limited availability of clinical psychologists, psychiatrists, and other specialist therapists, and negative or sceptical attitudes to such treatment. In addition, some of the outdated suspicions, embarrassment or fears about seeing a mental health professional persist as an obstacle to such referrals. Once engaged in cognitive–behavioural therapy, however, most patients do find it acceptable, credible, and helpful. Complications can arise from coexisting problems. In many cases the person is depressed as well as panicky, and this can interfere with treatment directly (due to lack of motivation, self-absorption, insomnia, lack of energy, or feelings of helplessness) or indirectly. Depressive thoughts and feelings may be tangled with the panic thoughts, both confusing and impeding progress. Marital or relationship problems can be a source of distress and confusion, obscuring the nature and the contributing causes of the panic disorder. Depending on the nature and seriousness of the coexisting problems, it may be necessary to deal with these before tackling the panics (such as reducing the depression), or arranging for the provision of marital counselling where necessary. Patients who are substance abusers can present special problems. For example, the progress of treatment of a patient with panic disorder and agoraphobia was impeded by intermittent bouts of excessive drinking that left him shaky and highly anxious.

When the panic disorder is associated with severe agoraphobia the patient may find it extremely difficult to travel to treatment. Energetic attempts need be made, directly or via friends/relatives or family doctor, to encourage the patient to attend, even if they have to be accompanied in the early stages. In the most severe, housebound cases, it may be necessary to begin the treatment in the patient's home. Such domiciliary work is extremely time-consuming and expensive, and may not be available from many clinics. Self-help treatment manuals and treatment advice by regular telephone contact are increasingly used by services, with some success.

Physical illnesses

If the panic disorder patient also has a significant physical illness, such as a cardiovascular disorder, or hypoglycaemia, this may complicate treatment. Some of the anti-panic medications may interact adversely with the patient's other medications and are to be avoided. Some illnesses can also complicate psychological treatment. For example, the patient's dizziness may be a symptom of some disorder of the ear, and not, or not always, a manifestation of anxiety. Similarly, the treatment of a panic patient who really does have a cardiac problem can be complicated. In these cases, the therapist will work closely with the family doctor and/or specialist physician. In a small but significant minority of cases, investigation for possible physical illness is crucial.

10 *Some practical advice*

• •

Is there a problem?

We all experience anxiety at one time or another, and a significant minority of the population experiences occasional episodes of panic. Most people are rarely concerned or worried about the occasional episode of panic, particularly if the cause of the panic is easily recognized and understandable, such as a near collision while driving. However, repeated episodes of severe panic, particularly those that come 'out of the blue', are distressing and troubling. They very often are associated with, or a direct cause of, significant anxiety about one's health. If you have high, continuing levels of anxiety and repeated episodes of panic, if your panics interfere with your life and activity (such as restricting your movements), then you need to consider seeking help.

Some key questions

At this stage you may need to ask yourself some questions about the problem, and the following ones may help to focus your attention:

- Are you having recurrent episodes of intense fear which arise rapidly and last for ten minutes or more?

- Are any of these episodes totally unexpected?

- Are these episodes of panic a source of considerable distress and concern?

- Have the panics generated serious anxiety about your health?

- Do you find yourself constantly avoiding certain activities, places, or people as a result of the panics?

- Has your job, or other occupations, become more difficult as a result of the panics?

- Are you concerned about the social effects of your panics, and are they a source of significant embarrassment for you?

- Are your panics a significant nuisance or hindrance to other people?

- Do you find yourself spending a great deal of time worrying about the episodes of panic and their possible meaning for your health?

If your answer to at least some of these questions is 'yes', then your anxiety and panic probably do require attention, and you may wish to consider taking action.

Concern about a member of the family

The same considerations apply when a spouse, relative, or friend observes a high level of anxiety, panic, and increasing avoidance behaviour in another person. If the affected person shows major changes in behaviour, and is becoming increasingly dependent on friends and relatives to get about to do the shopping or to travel to work, then the family may be justifiably worried. As mentioned earlier, daily or weekly fluctuations in the affected person's level of anxiety, tendency to have panics, and immobility can be a source of puzzlement in the family. If persistent difficulties are observed despite the fluctuations, the family needs to be concerned and take action.

In a small number of cases, the person attempts to conceal the true nature of their problem. In one example, a young married woman had fear of panics about going out on her own, but did not tell her family about this. She would go to great lengths to ensure that she always had someone with her when she went out of the house. When this was not possible, she would simply not go out, and give excuses ('I couldn't do the shopping today because I had a headache'). Eventually it emerged that unbeknownst to her husband she had been the victim of an attempted sexual molestation many years ago, which led to the panics. She did not wish to divulge this to her husband. When her avoidance of going out unaccompanied became obvious to the husband, he insisted on her getting help.

Seeking help

Once it is recognized that there is a problem, the best course of action is to seek professional advice. In some cases it may be possible to deal with the difficulties without much professional assistance, but in most cases seeking the advice of a qualified professional, at least in order to obtain a full assessment, is the best course of action.

Finding a therapist

The first step is to go to your own doctor and explain the problem as fully as possible, giving a complete and accurate account of the episodes of panic. You should also make a point of describing the effects on your behaviour, mobility, and social and occupational activities. As described on p. 50 above, your family doctor may well be able to help you deal with the problem, and be in a position to provide valuable education and reassurance. In a number of instances the doctor may prescribe appropriate medication as well.

However, if the problem is particularly severe or complex, or if you fail to derive significant benefit from the medication and other medical advice, your doctor may consider a referral to a specialist, usually a clinical psychologist or a psychiatrist. If you are referred to a psychiatrist they may decide to begin treatment with medication or, if there are good reasons not to take this course of action, you may be referred to a clinical psychologist who is trained in the use of the cognitive–behavioural therapy described in Chapter 6. A minority of psychiatrists are trained in this kind of work themselves, and they may give you this therapy without referring on. Sometimes, a referral may be made to a specialist nurse therapist with expertise in this kind of work.

In Britain, the local health service should be able to direct your doctor to a suitable therapist. If the doctor is unaware of a suitable local therapist, the British Association for Behavioural and Cognitive Psychotherapies (BABCP) can advise on therapists in each area. Most of the therapists work within the National Health Service in Britain, but if you prefer to see someone privately, the BABCP will be able to advise you, as will the organization called Psychology at Work Limited. General advice on the services of clinical psychologists and psychiatrists can be obtained from their respective professional organizations, the British Psychological Society and the Royal College of Psychiatrists. Advice is also obtainable from MIND, the National Association for Mental Health, and from various self-help organizations such as Phobic Action, No Panic, and First Steps to Freedom.

In the United States, health care provisions vary considerably from state to state, but most are well supplied with psychiatrists and clinical psychologists. Information about clinical psychologists who specialize in providing cognitive–behavioural therapy can be obtained from the American Psychological Association and from the Association for the Advancement of Behavior Therapy. In addition, a voluntary and non-profit organization called the Anxiety Disorders Association of America, provides useful information and advice about the disorder.

In Canada the clinical services vary from province to province, as do the health care insurance policies. In some provinces, psychological therapy is included as part of the comprehensive insurance policy, but in others, such as British Columbia, it is not. However, psychological treatment can be obtained at subsidized rates, or free, at some hospitals or university-associated clinics. Information about such services is generally available from the Psychological Association of each province or from the Canadian Psychological Association. Advice about psychiatric care can be obtained from the Canadian Psychiatric Association and from the provincial psychiatric associations. The Canadian Mental Health Association will also provide advice and information.

Addresses of the organizations mentioned above, and of a few other useful centres and agencies, are given in Appendix 4.

The therapist's assessment

When you go for your assessment, the therapist will try to collect as much relevant information as possible, and it may well take more than a single interview to complete the full assessment. The therapist is likely to request information described in the previous chapters, especially pp. 56–64. The therapist is also likely to ask you to complete some questionnaires, checklists, or other short tests. If your problem includes a significant amount of avoidance behaviour, these will probably be supplemented by a behavioural avoidance test, in which you will be asked to travel various distances while observed by the therapist (such as walk from the clinic entrance to the shops two blocks away). The therapist may ask you to keep a daily diary and record of your anxiety and/ or panics as they occur in the week or two following the initial assessment, like the ones shown in Figures 3 and 4 (see pp.

60–61). The therapist may wish to discuss the problem with a family member or close friend, subject to your agreement. If you are severely agoraphobic, verging on being housebound, it sometimes is necessary for the therapist to include a home visit as part of the assessment.

The planning and conduct of psychological therapy

In planning the treatment programme, your therapist will discuss with you the two main elements of treatment: the cognitive analysis and the behavioural exposure exercises. Nowadays, virtually all treatment of panic disorders is carried out on an out-patient basis, and hospitalization is rarely considered to be an option. Indeed, it is only in the most exceptional or complicated cases that admission to a hospital would be considered; even then it is likely to be for a very short period.

Throughout the therapy you are likely to be asked to keep regular records of your daily levels of anxiety, and the occurrence or non-occurrence of episodes of panic. You may also be asked to keep records of the strength of some of your panic-related beliefs (such as, 'I have panics because I have a weak heart'). The occurrence of particular stresses or unusual events may also be recorded. These recordings of your progress are important as they provide a good deal of continuous information, and the progress and modification of treatment is dependent largely on the completeness and accuracy of the information that is coming in. Relying on your recollection of various events that have taken place over a two- or four-week period is not a substitute for the daily recording of events as they occur. The records also serve a useful function in helping you to plot your progress, which usually is gradual and steady, and which in turn acts as a source of inspiration and encouragement for further efforts.

In some cases it might be necessary to have the active involvement of a relative or friend in the planning and conduct of the exposure exercises. However, in order to avoid any ambiguity which might lead to conflict within the family, the role that the relative plays should be clearly defined and detailed, with specific instructions and guidance provided by the therapist. It is also advisable for the relatives and friends to remember that the early progress which the patient makes is not a sign that the problem is entirely solved; sometimes relatives and friends become too eager and demanding for rapid progress. They should also be aware of the fluctuations in fear, panic, and avoidance referred to earlier, and that these fluctuations may persist for a time during the conduct of the therapy.

What you can do to facilitate the treatment

Psychological therapy for panic disorder is essentially a joint venture. The therapist can do very little without your active co-operation, because a large part of the treatment will depend upon your effort. To a considerable extent, the role of the therapist merges with that of an instructor or tutor, in which you are given the advice and direction in order to carry out the cognitive and behavioural changes that are necessary.

Both the cognitive and behavioural work can be distressing and difficult, and certainly fear-provoking at times. But if you are strongly motivated to overcome the problem, you will find that, with the help of the therapist, you can endure and persist until the problem is dealt with. Occasional returns of anxiety or even the occasional episode of panic should not be seen as a failure, and you should not allow yourself to be discouraged by them. Your improvement should be progressive and smooth, but do not be too surprised if there are some disappointments and some difficult days or even weeks. The beneficial effects are of lasting value in most cases.

As you gradually improve during the course of treatment you may well find that you have to readjust your behaviour. If you have been immobilized, partly or largely, by your panics and their consequences, you will need to re-establish your old ways of travel and mobility, and social and other contacts that had lapsed because of your difficulties. Members of your family will also have to make adjustments, and get used to the significant alterations in your behaviour. For example, they may need quite a few reminders before they recognize that they no longer have to accompany you on shopping expeditions, or ensure that someone is always in the house when you are at home. Your increasing independence will have major effects on the lives of your family members, and on their relationship with you. The family of one patient, who had been severely affected by panic disorder and related restrictions in mobility, and who improved considerably after treatment said: 'Our life has completely changed. We live normally once again'.

After therapy

When you have achieved significant improvement, do not expect to be totally free of anxiety. It often happens that the episodes of panic decrease or stop altogether, and the frightening thoughts that accompany them also wane. However, some of the thoughts may linger on in a milder fashion at the back of your mind, and you may feel that you are not absolutely free of them. Try to remember that anxiety is a universal experience, and that a very occasional episode of panic need not signify the return of a significant problem. Many people have occasional episodes of panic and yet live a perfectly normal and full life.

Once successfully treated, the chances of a major relapse are not very high. There may, however, be occasional lapses in which you sense a return of the urge to avoid situations formerly associated with panic. You should try to resist the return of avoidance behaviour even if it is difficult to do so at the time, because it can become the source of a return of fear. In fact, it is best to regard the return of even mild urges to avoid as a sure sign that you need to re-introduce some of the exposure exercises that you originally completed during treatment. This is the best way of giving yourself protection against a return of the problem. If, however, you do experience more than one severe episode of panic, you should return to the therapist for further advice, and possibly for a few booster treatments. These tend to be highly effective, and it is unusual for a successfully treated patient ever to require a second full course of treatment. Many therapists ask their patients to return after several months, anyway, to check on progress and arrange for booster sessions if necessary.

Self-treatment

If your problem is not very severe, and if there are no other complications, it may be possible for you to complete the treat-ment without professional assistance. If you have other psychological problems, especially depression, it is unwise to attempt a course of self-treatment, and you would do well to seek professional advice early on. If you habitually use a good deal of alcohol or drugs, such as benzodiazepines, self-help should not be attempted without first consulting your doctor. Or, if the episodes of panic are associated with distressing and troubling thoughts about your health, or even your life, then the assistance of a professional should be sought. The problem that lends itself most directly to self-treatment is avoidance. You should select a small number of clearly defined behavioural targets that you wish to achieve, such as walk to the local post office and back; walk round the block at a quiet time; go to the nearest supermarket for a short time, and so on. It is sensible to start with a fairly easy goal initially and then, as you begin to make progress walking or driving towards the goal, you can become more ambitious and expand your targets to include more distant and more difficult targets. It is advisable to carry out these self-exposure exercises on a regular basis, otherwise you run the risk of losing some of the benefits during the long intervals in between.

It sometimes is helpful to have a relative or friend monitor your progress and plan the next targets on your list. Whether you work entirely on your own, or with the assistance of a friend or relative, you will find it extremely helpful to keep good records of your progress. They will make it easier for you to plan your targets and to identify any difficulties that may arise; you can use a form similar to the one that is shown in Figures 7 and 8. If you tend to be generally anxious, or you find that you are getting exceedingly anxious during the exercises, a useful addition to your self-treatment programme is training in relaxation and breathing retraining. A brief guide to these methods is provided in Appendix 3 and on pp. 54–55 respectively. You should be sure to find the time to practise regularly. You can use the relaxation and breathing exercises before you set out on an exposure exercise, during the exercise if you begin to feel tense or anxious, and as a way of reducing anxiety and tension at other times.

A word of caution

A word of caution is needed about self-treatment. It is not advisable to undertake treatment entirely on your own unless your problems are relatively straightforward and consist mainly of avoidance behaviour. Even if you carry out much or most of the therapy entirely by yourself, it is often useful to discuss your problems at the outset with a qualified therapist. The therapist will be able to advise you

---

Date:

Target:

Time:

Alone or accompanied:

If accompanied, by whom:

Anxiety (0–100) — Before:
                        During (highest):
                        After:

Any panics:

Comments:

Figure 7 A blank example of a record sheet for an exposure session.

about whether or not a self-therapy programme is suitable and likely to be effective, and may also agree to monitor your progress from time to time. For people who do not have easy access to a therapist, a self-treatment programme may be the only option, but even here, an initial assessment and some form of monitoring, even by telephone, is advisable.

Date:	7th May
Target:	Buy something in supermarket
Time:	3 p.m.
Alone or accompanied:	Accompanied
If accompanied, by whom:	Bob (my husband)
Anxiety (0–100) — Before:	30
During (highest):	70
After:	20
Any panics:	None
Comments:	Felt quite anxious going in, as it was very crowded. Held Bob's hand when we entered. Picked up a few things quickly, it wasn't too bad then. Felt anxious again while waiting to pay at the check-out. Having Bob near me helped. He kept talking to me. Felt good when we came out.

Figure 8 A completed example of a record sheet for an exposure session.

A word of hope

Remember that episodes of panic are experienced by many, and are not a sign of something sinister. Panic disorder, even when it is quite severe and handicapping, is a treatable condition. With the right advice, appropriate therapy, and your own effort, it can be overcome. Many, many people have done so.

11 *Some common questions*

Is panic disorder a mental illness?

Panic disorder is a psychological problem and is not related to schizophrenia, mania, or any other major mental illness. People who experience recurrent episodes of panic are not insane and nor are they going to go insane. Panic disorder is a problem of anxiety, and has nothing to do with insanity as that term is broadly used.

Will my children inherit panic disorder?

Panic disorder, as such, is not inherited; there is, however, evidence of the inheritance of a predisposition to experience excessive anxiety, which is probably more common among relatives of people with panic disorder. A predisposition does not mean that someone will necessarily develop the disorder in question. As a group, the first-degree relatives (parents, children, brothers, sisters) of a person with panic disorder are more likely than the average to experience a similar disorder at some time in their lives. These are, however, group averages and it is not possible to predict exactly who will and who will not experience problems.

Should I conceal the fact that I have panic disorder?

There is no good reason to conceal it, and certainly no reason for embarrassment or shame. It remains true that there is a lot of ignorance about panic disorder and other psychological problems, despite some useful progress in public education, and ill-informed people may misunderstand the nature of your difficulties. The decision to enlighten them rests with you. Close friends and relatives tend to be more sympathetic and understanding and, in almost all instances, it is best to speak openly about your anxiety and the associated problems. You certainly should feel free to discuss your feelings fully with your doctor.

In some circumstances, ill-advised employers may be prejudiced against a person with a panic disorder, and this is one of the few times, perhaps the only one, in which discretion may be needed.

If you wish to speak about your panic disorder outside of therapy, and also wish to listen to the experiences of other people, you may do well to join one of the many self-help groups that have been formed over the past few years.

Some useful addresses are provided in Appendix 4. If there is no such organization in your area, you may even consider starting one.

Will my children start to imitate my panics?

This is extremely unlikely. Depending on age, your children will be aware of days and times when you appear to be tense and/or anxious. If your symptoms are severe and frequent they are likely to be concerned about you and may even acquire anxiety themselves. However, it is improbable that they will display episodes of panic, even if they observe you experiencing panics on occasion.

What is the long-term outlook for panic disorder?

At present we have insufficient information about the natural (that is, untreated) course of panic disorder, but in agoraphobia, up to one-third of all people experience spontaneous improvement within two years of the onset of the problem. Descriptions given by panic disorder patients suggest that the course of the untreated disorder is a fluctuating one in many cases. But these accounts are retrospective, and may be inaccurate The main reason for our ignorance about the untreated course of panic disorder is that the problem is now readily diagnosed, and effective treatments are available. On current evidence, which is sparse but accumulating, the long-term outlook after successful cognitive–behavioural therapy is highly favourable. Relatively few relapses have been recorded.

Even after successful treatment, however, a recurrence of stress, the onset of depression, or suffering a traumatic event, can result in a partial return of the problem. In these cases, a short course of booster treatments may be required.

With some of the medications, notably benzodiazepines, relapse can be a major problem when the drugs are stopped. In order to reduce the prospect of a relapse, the medications should be tapered off very gradually, under medical supervision.

What is the effect of repeated episodes of panic?

Many patients worry that the effects of their episodes of panic may be cumulative, as in 'Can my body stand the repeated strain'? The recurrent panics generate a great deal of anxiety and worry, and frequently lead to changes in behaviour and lifestyle, but there is no evidence that recurrent panics cause any damage to one's health. The damage, such as it is, appears to be purely psychological, which is dealt with in therapy.

How can I reduce the side-effects of the medications?

Most medications that produce beneficial therapeutic effects are also prone to produce some unwanted side-effects. The most common side-effects for the main anti-panic medications are set out on pp. 31–33. There are wide individual differences in the occurrence of side-effects, and it is difficult to predict exactly what to expect for each patient—some patients can tolerate one type of medication but react badly to another. As a result, the search for the correct medication, and the most effective, tolerable dose for the particular patient, may require patience. Your doctor will discuss in advance the possible side-effects of your medication with you, and you must keep the doctor in the picture about the side-effects that you experience. Fortunately, most patients find that they gradually become accustomed to the side-effects and worry less about them as the benefits of treatment become evident.

Can hypnosis cure panic attacks?

Claims are often made by various people, including hypnotists, that they can 'cure' episodes of panic quickly. In hypnotherapy, the person is brought to a trance-like state by suggestion, and in this state, they may be told that there will be no more panic attacks. Unfortunately, such post-hypnotic suggestions do not seem to produce lasting beneficial effects. The main problem with hypnosis, and other alternative therapies, is that they have not been properly evaluated, and what little evaluation that has been done has not produced good evidence of efficacy. This is in contrast to the treatments described in Chapters 6 and 7, which have been the subject of previous and ongoing research.

Is it true that drinking coffee can cause panic attacks?

Caffeine, which is present in many common drinks such as coffee, tea, cola and cocoa, does not cause panic disorder, but it can exacerbate panic symptoms. Caffeine has also been used in laboratory studies to induce panic attacks in patients with panic disorder. Many patients suffering from panic disorder learn to avoid caffeine, through experience. This does not mean that drinking coffee, or other beverages which contain caffeine, in moderation causes panic symptoms.

Appendix 1

• •

The Mobility Inventory

Please indicate the degree to which you avoid the following places or situations because of discomfort or anxiety. Rate your amount of avoidance when you are with a trusted companion and when you are alone. Do this by using the following scale.

1 = Never avoid

2 = Rarely avoid

3 = Avoid about half the time

4 = Avoid most of the time

5 = Always avoid

(You may use numbers halfway between those listed when you think it is appropriate. For example, 3½ or 4½).

Write your score in the blanks for each situation or place under both conditions: when accompanied, and, when alone. Leave blank those situations that do not apply to you.

Places	When accompanied	When alone
Theatres	_____	_____
Supermarkets	_____	_____
Classrooms	_____	_____
Department stores	_____	_____
Restaurants	_____	_____
Museums	_____	_____
Elevators	_____	_____
Auditoriums or stadiums	_____	_____
Parking garages	_____	_____
High places	_____	_____
Tell how high	_____	_____
Enclosed spaces		
(e.g. tunnels)	_____	_____

Open spaces
  (A) Outside (e.g. fields,
  wide streets, courtyards)   ————   ————
  (B) Inside (e.g. large
  rooms, lobbies)   ————   ————

Riding In

Buses	————	————
Trains	————	————
Subways	————	————
Airplanes	————	————
Boats	————	————

Driving or riding in car
  (A) At any time   ————   ————
  (B) On expressways   ————   ————

Situations

Standing in lines	————	————
Crossing bridges	————	————
Parties or social gatherings	————	————
Walking on the street	————	————
Staying at home alone	NA	————
Being far away from home	————	————
Other (specify)	————	————

We define a panic attack as:

(1) a high level of anxiety accompanied by

(2) strong body reactions (heart palpitations, sweating, muscle tremors, dizziness, nausea) with

(3) the temporary loss of the ability to plan, think, or reason and

(4) the intense desire to escape or flee the situation.
(Note: this is different from high anxiety or fear alone.)

Please indicate the total number of panic attacks you have had in the last 7 days.

————

From Chambless, Caputo, Jasin, Graceley, and Williams (1985). See p. 95 for reference. Reproduced with permission.

Appendix 2

The Cognitions Questionnaire

Below are some thoughts or ideas that may pass through your mind when you are nervous or frightened.

Please indicate how often each thought occurs when you are nervous.

Rate from 1–5 using the scale below:

1 = thought never occurs.

2 = thought rarely occurs.

3 = thought occurs during half of the times I am nervous.

4 = thought usually occurs.

5 = thought always occurs when I am nervous

Thought	*Rating*
I am going to be sick	_____
I am going to faint	_____
I must have a brain tumour	_____
I shall have a heart attack	_____
I shall choke to death	_____
I am going to act foolishly	_____
I am going blind	_____
I shall not be able to control myself	_____
I shall hurt someone	_____
I am going to have a stroke	_____
I am going to go insane	_____
I am going to scream	_____
I am going to babble or talk in a funny way	_____
I shall be paralyzed by fear	_____

OTHER IDEAS NOT LISTED (PLEASE DESCRIBE AND RATE THEM)
_____
_____

From Chambless, Caputo, Bright, and Gallagher (1984). See p. 95 for reference. Reproduced with permission.

Appendix 3

· ·

Learning to relax: a simple guide

Do your relaxation exercises in a quite room, at a time when you are not likely to be disturbed. Sit comfortably in an armchair. Make sure that your clothes are not tight. Remove belts, spectacles, and shoes.

Learn to relax by first tensing and then relaxing various muscle groups of the body, one at a time. Keep your eyes closed throughout. At each step, keep the muscles tensed, quite hard, for 6–8 seconds, and notice the tension. Concentrate on the muscles, and notice the tension. Then relax the muscles, and keep them relaxed for 45–50 seconds. Again, concentrate on the muscles, and notice how the feelings of relaxation differ from those of tension. You can learn to time yourself quite easily by slowly counting for the first few times. Remember to repeat the tense–relax cycle for each muscle group before you move on to the next. When you tense a group of muscles, take in a breath and hold it until you relax the muscles, and release the breath slowly as you relax.

Given below is the order in which to tense and relax the various muscle groups. For each muscle group, a strategy for making them tense is given. For some, alternative strategies are suggested. Before you actually start the proper relaxation exercises, learn the way in which each muscle group can be effectively tensed. Try out one at a time, and master it. Where alternatives are suggested, decide which one is going to be your regular strategy.

Once this is done, you can begin the actual sessions.

1. *Right hand and forearm*: Tense the muscles by making a tight first; or, try pressing the inner part of the finger tips against the base of the thumb. Relax by slowly opening the hand.

2. *Right biceps*: Tense the muscles by pushing your elbow into the arm of the chair, or by pressing the elbow and the upper arm into the side of the rib cage. Relax by returning to original position.

3. *Left hand and forearm*: As for right hand and forearm.

4. *Left biceps*: As for right biceps.

(*Note*: If you are left-handed, do steps 3 and 4 first, followed by steps 1 and 2.)

5. *Forehead*: Tense by raising your eyebrows as high as possible with your eyes still closed. Relax by returning eyebrows to normal position.

6. *Upper cheeks and nose*: Tense by squinting and screwing up your eyes, and wrinkling the nose. Relax by returning to normal state.

7. *Lower cheeks and jaws*: Tense by clenching your teeth together and pulling back the corners of your mouth. Relax by unclenching the teeth and bringing mouth back to normal.

8. *Neck*: Tense by pulling your chin into your chest, but not quite touching it. Relax by returning to original position.

9. *Shoulder and chest*: Tense by raising and pulling your shoulder blades towards each other. Relax by returning to original position.

10. *Stomach and abdomen*: Tense by pulling in your stomach and abdomen as much as you can. You can also tense these muscles by pushing out your stomach and abdomen. Relax by returning to original state.

11. *Right leg*: Tense by straightening the whole leg from the hip, parallel to the floor. Relax by lowering and resting the leg on the floor again.

12. *Right foot*: Tense by pushing your heel into the floor and curling your toes upwards—that is, towards you. Relax by returning to original position.

13. *Left leg*: As for right leg.

14. *Left foot*: As for right foot.

(*Note*: If your dominant leg is the left one, do steps 13 and 14 before 11 and 12.)

15. *Whole body*: Tense as many of the above muscle groups as you can all at once, making yourself into a 'ball of tension'. You will find that you can tense most of the muscle groups together; in fact, if you use the tension strategies suggested above, there will be only two of these items that you will not be able to do while doing everything else. One is the raising of the eyebrows, but the eyebrows can be tensed by wrinkling them when you screw up the eyes. The second is the pushing of your heels into the floor, but with your legs stretched, you will still be able to curl your toes up towards you.

Remember that each step is to be done twice, including the last 'all-body' step. Remember also to take in a breath and hold it when the muscles are kept tense, and to release the breath as you relax the muscles.

After the whole sequence is completed, continue to sit in a relaxed state for several minutes. At this point, you may imagine a pleasant scene, like a peaceful beach or a flower garden. With practice, when you become more skilled in relaxing yourself, you will find that the exercises become quite easy. After some weeks of practice, you will be able to relax yourself by simply tensing and relaxing the entire body—that is, the last step of the sequence given above—without going through the separate steps. With even more practice, many people acquire the ability to relax very effectively simply by concentrating on making their muscles relaxed without having first to tense them.

If you prefer to do your relaxation exercises lying down on a bed or the floor, only minor changes to the above programme are needed. For each leg, what you will need to do is to raise it from the bed or floor to form an angle of about 30 degrees. Relax by lowering and resting the leg on the bed or floor.

There is no particular time of the day when relaxation should be practised, but avoid doing it when you are very sleepy, to avoid falling asleep while relaxing. Try to do it daily in the early stages, so you will quickly become good at it.

There are different sequences of muscle groups suggested by different authors for relaxation exercises. There is no particular advantage of one over the others. What is important is to use a sequence which is fairly logical, as the one given here, not a random or haphazard one. You should use the same sequence regularly, so it will be easier to learn and master it.

There are cassette tapes available commercially which give recorded instructions for relaxation training. Using one of these can be useful in the early stages, but it is important to wean yourself gradually away from the cassette, as the aim is to learn to relax without any external aid. The following are some good cassettes that are commercially available:

Robert Sharpe's cassette *Relax and enjoy it*, which is available from Aleph One Ltd, The Old Courthouse, High Street, Bottisham, Cambridge CB5 9BA.

Jane Madders's cassette *Self-help relaxation*, available from Relaxation for Living Ltd, 29 Burwood Park Road, Walton-on-Thames, Surrey KT12 5LH.

Roy Bailey's cassette *Systematic relaxation pack*, which comes with a booklet, produced by Winslow Press Ltd, 9 London Lane, London E8 3PR.

The relaxation cassette produced by First Steps to Freedom, 22 Randall Road, Kenilworth, Warwickshire CV8 1JY.

Appendix 4

Addresses of useful organizations

UK

British Association for Behavioural
and Cognitive Psychotherapies
c/o Harrow Psychological Health
Services
Northwick Park Hospital
Watford Road
Harrow
Middlesex HA1 3UJ

British Psychological Society
48 Princess Road East
Leicester LE1 7DR

Royal College of Psychiatrists
17 Belgrave Square
London SW1X 8PG

MIND, National Association for
Mental Health
22 Harley Street
London W1N 2ED

Psychology at Work Ltd
155 Regents Park Road
London NW1 8BB

First Steps to Freedom
22 Randall Road
Kenilworth
Warwickshire CV8 1JY

No Panic
93 Brands Farm Way
Raudlay
Telford TF3 2JQ

Open Door Association
447 Pensby Road
Heswall
Merseyside L61 9PQ

Phobic Action
Hornbeam House
Claybury Grounds
Manor Road
Woodford Green
Essex 1G8 8PR

Phobics Society
4 Cheltenham Road
Chorlton-cum-Hardy
Manchester M21 1QN

USA

Association for Advancement of
Behavior Therapy
305 Seventh Avenue
New York, NY 10001

American Psychiatric Association
1400 K Street, NW
Washington, DC 20005

American Psychological Association
750 First Street, NE
Washington, DC 20002–4242

The Anxiety Disorders Association
of America
6000 Executive Boulevard
Suite 2000
Rockville, Maryland 20852–3801

CANADA

Canadian Psychiatric Association
Suite 200
237 Argyle Avenue
Ottawa
Ontario
K2P 1B8

Canadian Psychological Association
Vincent Road
Old Chelsea
Quebec
JOX 2NO

Canadian Mental Health Association
65 Brunswick Street
Fredericton
New Brunswick E3B 1G5

Appendix 5

•••••••••••••••••••••••••••••••••••••••

Some useful reading

Technical

There are several major books that cover the topic of panic disorder. These include:

Wolfe, B. E. and Maser, J. D. (ed.) (1994) *Treatment of panic disorder*. American Psychiatric Press, Washington, DC, USA.
   This book, which reports the proceedings of a major Consensus Development Conference, is strong on pharmacological and psychological treatments.
Rachman, S. and Maser, J. D. (ed.) (1988) *Panic: psychological perspectives*. Lawrence Erlbaum, Hillsdale, NJ, USA.
   This gives a presentation of facts, theories, and commentaries of leading authorities. It is particularly useful for those interested in theoretical accounts.
McNally, R.J. (1994) *Panic disorder: a critical analysis*. Guilford Press, New York, USA.
   A thorough and critical analysis of all aspects of panic disorder.
Barlow, D. H. (1988) *Anxiety and its disorders*. Guilford Press, New York, USA.
   An excellent book on the whole range of anxiety disorders.

For briefer accounts, see:
Clark, D. M. (1989) Anxiety states: panic and generalized anxiety. In *Cognitive behaviour therapy for psychiatric problems: a practical guide* (ed. K. Hawton, P. Salkovskis, J. Kirk and D. M. Clark), pp. 52–96. Oxford University Press, Oxford.
   Excellent account of cognitive–behavioural treatment.
Craske, M. G. and Barlow, D. H. (1993) Panic disorder and agoraphobia. In *Clinical handbook of psychological disorders (2nd edn)* (ed. D. H. Barlow), pp. 1–47. Guilford Press, New York, USA.
   Another excellent and up-to-date account of psychological treatment.

For a review of relaxation techniques and their efficacy, see:
Lichstein, K. (1988) *Clinical relaxation strategies*. Wiley, New York, USA.

Readers who wish to consult the original papers by the main contributors to the debate about the theory of panic disorder might find the following helpful:

Clark, D.M. (1986). A cognitive approach to panic. *Behaviour Research and Therapy*, **24**, pp. 461–70.

Clark, D.M. (1988). A cognitive model of panic attacks. In *Panic: psychological perspectives* (ed. S. Rachman and J.D. Maser), pp. 71–89. Lawrence Erlbaum, Hillsdale, NJ, USA.

Klein, D.F. (1964). Delineation of two drug-responsive anxiety syndromes. *Psychopharmacologia*, **5**, pp.397–408.

Klein, D.F. (1993). False suffocation alarms, spontaneous panics, and related conditions: an integrative hypothesis. *Archives of General Psychiatry*, **50**, pp.306–17.

Klein, D.F. and Klein, H.M. (1989). The definition and psychopharmacology of spontaneous panic and phobia. In *Psychopharmacology of anxiety* (ed. P. Tyrer), pp. 135–62. Oxford University Press, New York, USA.

Klein, D.F. and Klein, H.M. (1989). The nosology, genetics, and theory of spontaneous panic and phobia. In *Psychopharmacology of anxiety, op.cit.*, pp. 163–95.

A useful evaluation of the efficacy of different treatment approaches is found in:

Gould, R.A., Otto, M.W. and Pollack, M.H. (1995). A meta-analysis of treatment outcome for panic disorder. *Clinical Psychology Review*, **15**, pp. 819–44.

Non-technical

Useful accounts, including practical advice, are found in the following:

Seligman, M.E.P. (1994) *What you can change and what you can't*. Knopf, New York, USA.

Clear, balanced and up-to-date account of psychological problems and treatment, including a chapter on panic disorder, by an expert clinical researcher.

Ingham, C. (1993) *Panic attacks: what they are, why they happen, and what you can do about them*. Thorsons, London.

A readable and detailed guide, written by someone who has herself suffered from panic.

Barlow, D.H. and Craske, M.G. (1989) *Mastery of your anxiety and panic*. Graywind, Albany, USA.

A most useful account and advice by two acknowledged experts.

For an account of a related anxiety disorder, see:

de Silva, P. and Rachman, S. (1992) *Obsessive–compulsive disorder: the facts*. Oxford University Press, Oxford.

Appendix 6

. . . .

References cited in the text

American Psychiatric Association (1994) *Diagnostic and statistical manual of mental disorders*, (4th edn.) APA, Washington, DC, USA.

Barlow, D. H. and Craske, M. G. (1988) The phenomenology of panic. In *Panic: psychological perspectives* (ed. S. Rachman and J. D. Maser), pp. 11–35. Lawrence Erlbaum, Hillsdale, NJ, USA.

Chambless, D. L., Caputo, G. C., Bright, P., and Gallagher, R. (1984) Assessment of fear of fear in agorphobics: the Body Sensations Questionnaire and the Agoraphobic Cognitions Questionnaire. *Journal of Consulting and Clinical Psychology*, **52**, 1090–7.

Chambless, D. L., Caputo, G. C., Jasin, S. E., Gracely, E. J., and Williams, C. (1985). The Mobility Inventory for agoraphobia. *Behaviour Research and Therapy*, **23**, 35–44.

Clark, D. M. (1986). A cognitive approach to panic. *Behaviour Research and Therapy*, **24**, 461–70.

Clark, D. M. (1989). Anxiety states: panic and generalized anxiety. In *Cognitive behaviour therapy for psychiatric problems: a practical guide* (ed. K. Hawton, P.M. Salkovskis, J. Kirk and D. M. Clark), pp. 52–96. Oxford University Press, Oxford.

Wolfe, B. E. and Maser, J. D. (1994). *Treatment of panic disorder*. American Psychiatric Press, Washington, DC, USA.

Index